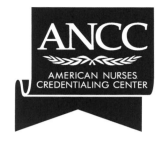

Magnet®: The Next Generation—Nurses Making the Difference

Magnet Recognition Program®

By Karen Drenkard, PhD, RN, NEA-BC, FAAN
   Gail Wolf, PhD, RN, FAAN
   Shirley H. Morgan, MSN, RN, NEA-BC

American Nurses Credentialing Center
Silver Spring, Maryland
2011

Library of Congress Cataloging-in-Publication Data
Magnet : the next generation : nurses making the difference / editors, Karen Drenkard, Gail A. Wolf, Shirley H. Morgan.
p. ; cm.
Includes bibliographical references and index.
ISBN 978-1-935213-48-2 (softcover)

1. Nursing—United States. 2. American Nurses Credentialing Center. Magnet Recognition Program. I. Drenkard, Karen. II. Wolf, Gail A. III. Morgan, Shirley H. IV. American Nurses Credentialing Center.

[DNLM: 1. American Nurses Credentialing Center. Magnet Recognition Program. 2. Nursing—organization & administration. 3. Leadership. 4. Models, Organizational. 5. Nursing Service, Hospital—standards. 6. Quality Assurance, Health Care—methods. 7. Quality Assurance, Health Care—organization & administration. WY 105]

RT4.M315 2010 610.73—dc22   2010044377

ISBN-13: 978-1-935213-48-2

First printing, December 2010

American Nurses Credentialing Center
8515 Georgia Ave., Suite 400
Silver Spring, MD 20910
1.800.284.2378
301.628.5000 tel 301.628.5004 fax
www.nursecredentialing.org

Contents

Magnet®: The Next Generation— Nurses Making the Difference

FOREWORD

Magnet: The Next Generation is the story of a remarkable journey—one that began more than 25 years ago when a group of visionary researchers set out to determine the reasons for the recurring nursing shortages plaguing our country. The researchers took an innovative approach. Rather than spend time chronicling what was wrong at hospitals with high nurse turnover, they focused on what was right at hospitals where RN vacancy and turnover were low. Their groundbreaking findings led to the creation of ANCC's Magnet Recognition Program® in 1990.

As we mark Magnet's 20th anniversary in 2010, we celebrate more than just a milestone. The program has made a profound impact on nursing and patient care in the United States and around the world. Each year, more and more hospitals embark on the Journey to Magnet Excellence™. They recognize that embracing and adopting Magnet® standards will create a safe, high-quality environment where their entire healthcare team can thrive. And they understand the importance of moving beyond quick fixes to focus on implementing long-term, sustainable structures and processes that will attract RNs and improve patient care.

In 2008, after intensive evaluation and analysis, the Magnet Recognition Program introduced its dynamic new model, which provides a framework for the next generation of nursing practice and research. The simpler format reflects a new emphasis on measuring outcomes, offers greater clarity and direction, eliminates redundancy, and serves as a roadmap for organizations seeking to achieve Magnet recognition.

Magnet: The Next Generation examines the evolution of the new model, taking an in-depth look at the rationale, structure, and intended outcomes of the five key components: Transformational Leadership; Structural Empowerment; Exemplary Professional Practice; New Knowledge, Innovations, and Improvements; and Empirical Outcomes.

It also explores the vast changes that have occurred since ANCC published its last book about the Magnet Recognition Program in 2002. These changes include global expansion of the Magnet program, the growing business case for Magnet recognition, key research supporting evidence of excellence, new challenges associated with caring for an aging population with chronic disease, and implications for future health policy.

Debbie D. Hatmaker, PhD, RN-BC, SANE-A
President, American Nurses Credentialing Center

PREFACE

It's hard to believe that 16 years have passed since the American Nurses Credentialing Center (ANCC) designated the University of Washington Medical Center as the first Magnet® recognized hospital in the United States.

Since then, ANCC's Magnet Recognition Program® has grown to include 377 healthcare organizations and hospitals around the country and the world. In just two decades, it has become the international gold standard for nursing excellence and outstanding patient care.

Magnet: The Next Generation chronicles this remarkable evolution, culminating in the transition to the new Magnet Model in 2008. It takes an in-depth look at the model's five major components and offers a framework for the next generation of nursing practice and research. Chapters focus on the structure, processes, and outcomes that nurses and nurse leaders will need to successfully navigate an ever-changing and ever more complex healthcare environment moving forward.

Whether you are part of a Magnet organization, on the Magnet journey, or considering taking the Journey to Magnet Excellence™, you'll find information about new standards, new paradigms, and new ways of delivering the best care for your patients.

Magnet: The Next Generation shares reflections and presents evidence as it explores what it means to be a part of a community of Magnet hospitals poised to meet the next generation of healthcare challenges. It is must reading for anyone who cares about nursing excellence, quality and safety, and the future of healthcare delivery in the United States and around the world.

Karen Drenkard, PhD, RN, NEA-BC, FAAN
Director, Magnet Recognition Program

Gail Wolf, PhD, RN, FAAN
Chair, Commission on Magnet Recognition

Acknowledgments

The editors would like to acknowledge the original researchers, whose ground-breaking research led to answers about nursing practice and the environment of excellence that shaped the Magnet Recognition Program®:
- Margaret L. McClure, EdD, RN, FAAN
- Muriel A. Poulin, EdD, RN, FAAN
- Margaret D. Sovie, PhD, RN, FAAN
- Mabel A. Wandelt, PhD, RN, FAAN.

The editors would like to thank the staff and leadership of the American Nurses Credentialing Center and the staff of the Magnet Recognition Program who provided support, research, and review of the manuscript. A special thanks to Shirley Morgan, MSN, RN, NEA-BC, assistant director, Magnet Recognition Program, who served as the lead reviewer through many months of edits.

The editors would like to thank the American Academy of Nursing and the American Nurses Association for the leadership and vision in creating the Magnet Recognition Program, and the American Nurses Credentialing Center's Boards and past presidents for their continued support.

The editors would like to thank the Commission on Magnet for their vision in creating this book to capture the history and future of nursing.

The editors would like to thank and recognize all of our contributing authors.

And finally, the editors would like to thank the community of Magnet Hospitals, who are doing the hard work of reaching a high bar of practice every day. Their work is truly amazing. As a result of their efforts, patient care is improving. They exemplify the "best of the best" in nursing care, and we cannot begin to thank them for all that they are doing to serve the most vulnerable among us: hospitalized patients in need of healing. We thank them for their commitment, dedication, and transformational leadership.

About the Authors

Mary Jo Assi, MS, RN, APRN-BC, AHN-BC

Mary Jo Assi is the Director of Advanced Practice Nursing at the Valley Hospital in Ridgewood, NJ. In that capacity, she has developed numerous APN clinical programs and services over the past 10 years. A graduate of the Englewood Hospital School of Nursing, she received her BSN from St. Louis University and a master's degree as a Family Nurse Practitioner from Pace University. She is currently pursuing her DNP at George Washington University. She has served on the Commission on Magnet for the past two years and represents the advanced practice nurse interest. She is a member of the American Academy of Nurse Practitioners, the American College of Nurse Practitioners, and Sigma Theta Tau.

Angela Creta, MS, RN, CNL-BC

Angela Creta is the Magnet Site Coordinator at the Miriam Hospital in Providence, RI. Angela was appointed to the Commission on Magnet in 2008 to represent the staff nurse perspective. Angela received her bachelor's and master's degrees from the University of Rhode Island. In her graduate work she participated in one of the nation's first clinical nurse leader partnerships. Angela is active with the Rhode Island State Nurses Association, serving as a peer reviewer of continuing education programs, and is an elected member of the Cabinet of Nursing Practice.

Karen Drenkard, PhD, RN, NEA-BC, FAAN

Karen Drenkard most recently served as the Senior Vice President, Nursing/Chief Nursing Executive at Inova Health Systems in Falls Church, VA. For the past eight years she has been responsible for nursing practice, education, research, strategy, and operations across one of Washington, DC's largest healthcare systems. With more than 3,900 nurses and multiple service sites, Dr. Drenkard had oversight of the nursing leadership team and the implementation of the vision for nursing services throughout the system.

During her tenure at Inova, she led two hospitals to successful Magnet designation and served as a champion of the program. She has published and presented extensively on the Magnet Recognition Program. In addition, Dr. Drenkard has been widely recognized for leadership, including being the recipient of prestigious awards from *Nursing Spectrum* (Nurse of the Year 2005, Advancing the Profession) and the American Organization of Nurse Executives (Executive Nurse Scholar of the Year 2005).

Dr. Drenkard earned her PhD in Nursing with a focus on administration, policy, and leadership from George Mason University in Fairfax, VA, and an MSN from Marymount University in Arlington, VA. Her experience includes significant teaching and research. She is a member of the National Advisory Council on Nurse Education and Practice, served on Virginia's Health Reform Commission, and served as the chair of the (Virginia) Governor's Advisory Council on the Future of Nursing. She is ANCC board certified as a Nurse Executive, Advanced.

Stephanie L. Ferguson, PhD, RN, FAAN

Stephanie Ferguson is an International Health Care Consultant for the American Nurses Credentialing Center. She is also Consulting Associate Professor for Stanford University in the Bing Stanford in Washington Program, Associate Professor and Coordinator of the Community Nursing Organization at the Virginia Commonwealth University School of Nursing, and Professor of Nursing at Lynchburg College. She consults widely with a variety of organizations and associations, such as the World Health Organization in her own private practice. Dr. Ferguson was the Director of the Leadership for Change Programme™ and Consultant for Nursing and Health Policy for the International Council of Nurses in Geneva, Switzerland. She served as a White House Fellow from 1996 to 1997, working for the President and the Secretary of Health and Human Services. She was appointed a member of the National Institute for Nursing Research, and she served as a member of the Board of Directors for the Bon Secours Health System, Inc., and member of the Board of Trustees for the Catholic Health Association. Currently, she is a Trustee for the Catholic Medical Mission Board. Dr. Ferguson has authored many publications and received numerous awards for her work in leadership and health policy development, health systems strengthening, and global health from a variety of organizations.

Jeanne Floyd, PhD, RN, CAE

Jeanne Floyd, certified in association management, has provided management services for a variety of nursing organizations, including the Pennsylvania State Nurses Association, the Midwest Alliance in Nursing, and Sigma Theta Tau International. For nine years, she has been the executive director of the American Nurses Credentialing Center. Her areas of expertise are strategic thinking and planning, organizational capacity building, volunteer and staff leadership development, and community building.

Dr. Floyd has invited internationally known healthcare leaders to develop the preferred future of ANCC through participation in think tanks and councils that have addressed certification, accreditation, the Magnet Recognition Program, the community of Magnet chief nurse officers, technology, credentialing research, strategic thinking, and international outreach. In tandem, extensive marketing and business operations surveys have been completed.

All of this has served to prepare ANCC to live out its mission to promote excellence in nursing and health care globally through credentialing programs and related services. As an example, the Magnet Recognition Program, with 377 recognized facilities, has approached the global tipping point for creating cultural attributes within healthcare systems that attract and retain competent nurses interested in joining interdisciplinary teams that seek to raise the bar for the provision of quality patient care. Through international outreach, partnerships are being created with nurse leaders around the world, especially in New Zealand, Australia, Singapore, and Lebanon.

Janet Y. Harris, MSN, RN, NEA-BC

Janet Harris has 36 years of nursing experience. She served as a charge nurse, head nurse, assistant director of nursing, faculty member, and associate hospital director in her early years. Currently, Janet serves as System Nurse Executive and CNO for the adult hospital and as interim CNO for the Batson Children's Hospital at the University of Mississippi Healthcare.

Janet served for four years on the Congress of Nursing Practice and Economics of the ANA and represented the group as a member of the Commission on Magnet Recognition with ANCC. She is a past President of the Mississippi Nurses Association and has been active in AONE over the years. She has numerous awards to her credit, including Mississippi Top 50 Businesswomen, Alumnus of the Decade (1980s) for the UMC School of Nursing, and the Nurse Executive Recognition Award from the Mississippi Hospital Association.

Joanne V. Hickey, PhD, APRN-BC, ACNP, FAAN, FCCM

Joanne Hickey is the Patricia L. Starck/PARTNERS Professor of Nursing at the University of Texas Health Science Center in Houston, School of Nursing. She is Director of the Doctor of Nursing Program and is an acute care nurse practitioner who has focused on neuroscience practice, publication, and research. She is a fellow of the American Academy of Nursing and the American College of Critical Care Medicine. Dr. Hickey is currently chairperson of the Research Council of the Institute for Credentialing Research at ANCC. The Research Council is focused on promoting credentialing research and supporting its dissemination. Dr. Hickey has also served on the ANCC Board of Directors and as chairperson of the Commission on Certification.

Christina Joy, DNSc, RN

Christina Joy is a member of the Magnet Program Office as a Senior Analyst at the American Nurses Credentialing Center. Dr. Joy is retired from the Navy Nurse Corps and has served in a number of clinical, managerial, and academic positions during her career. In her current position, she works with organizations pursuing Magnet designation.

Yasmin Kazzaz, MHA

Yasmin Kazzaz has extensive experience in complex academic health centers, including the University of Pittsburgh Medical Center, Pittsburgh, PA; the University of Texas M.D. Anderson Cancer Center, Houston, TX; Beth Israel Deaconess Medical Center, Boston, MA; and Methodist Health Care System, Houston, TX. Mrs. Kazzaz's contributions to health care have been in recruitment, advertising, and marketing; new program development; organizational development; academic–service partnerships; physician practice management; leadership development; and Magnet® readiness. Mrs. Kazzaz obtained her BS degree in Psychology from the University of Houston, Texas, and her Master's Degree in Health Care Administration from Washington University School of Medicine's Health Administration Program, St. Louis, MO. She serves health care as a Commissioner for the American Nurses Credentialing Center's Magnet Recognition Program®, representing the public. Yasmin has presented and been published at the national level.

Brenda Kelly, MA, RN, NEA-BC

Brenda Kelly is the Director of Nursing and Director of the Behavioral Health Service Line at North Carolina Baptist Hospital of Wake Forest University Baptist Medical Center in Winston-Salem, NC, where she is responsible for the implementation and coordination of care using a seamless delivery system providing easily accessible, cost-effective, high-quality care to patients. With experience in a variety of administrative roles at Wake Forest, she represented the patient care manager on the Commission on Magnet. She served as a member of the Commission from 2001 to 2009. Four of her years of service were as the Commission Chair. She oversaw exponential program growth and a comprehensive evaluation of the program to create the paradigm shift in the program we see today. She earned her graduate degree from Appalachian State University in Boone, NC, and her undergraduate degree from Lenoir-Rhyne College in Hickory, NC.

Lois L. Kercher, PhD, RN

Lois Kercher is an executive nurse leader in southeastern Virginia for Sentara Healthcare, where she served as Vice President for Nursing and System Chief Nursing Officer for six years. Her contribution to the understanding of nursing's role in patient safety has been recognized by her peers and colleagues. Dr. Kercher led Sentara Norfolk General Hospital's journey to achieve Magnet recognition status. She was the President of the American Organization of Nurse Executives (AONE) in 2000. She has been a member of the Commission on Magnet since 2004, representing AONE.

Vicki A. Lundmark, PhD

Vicki Lundmark has been the Director of the Institute for Credentialing Research of the American Nurses Credentialing Center since 2005. She holds a PhD in sociology from the University of Minnesota, with a graduate minor from the Center for Advanced Feminist Studies. Her major areas of interest are social stratification, women's work, and women's professions. Dr. Lundmark is the author of "Magnet environments for professional nursing practice," a literature review published in 2008 by the Agency for Healthcare Research and Quality in *Patient Safety and Quality: An Evidence-Based Handbook for Nurses.*

Rosemary Luquire, PhD, RN, NEA-BC, FAAN

Rosemary Luquire joined the Baylor Health Care System as Senior Vice President and Corporate Chief Nursing Officer in January 2007, responsible for overseeing nursing practice across 15 facilities representing 5000 nurses. Dr. Luquire joined Baylor from St. Luke's Episcopal Health System in Houston where she served as Senior Vice President, Chief Nursing Officer, and Chief Quality Officer. She was responsible for overseeing the healthcare system's professional nursing practice and the quality improvement program. In her 20 years at St. Luke's, Dr. Luquire earned a reputation for research-based practice, minimal staff turnover, and an unfailing commitment to cost-effective operations and patient care.

At Baylor, Dr. Luquire works as a member of the senior executive team, representing nursing across the system. She directs and facilitates system nursing policies, procedures, and standards of nursing practice to provide the highest quality of patient care. Dr. Luquire directs her energies toward the promotion and development of nursing as an ideal vocation and career opportunity.

A graduate of Emory University, Dr. Luquire earned her PhD from Texas Woman's University (TWU) and her master's degree in nursing from the University of Texas Health Science Center at Houston (UT). Dr. Luquire holds joint faculty appointments at both TWU and UT. She is a Fellow in the American Academy of Nursing; a commissioner for the Commission on Magnet in Silver Spring, MD, and a member of the American Nurses Association, the American Association of Critical-Care Nurses, and the national and local chapters of the American College of Healthcare Executives. Dr. Luquire has published extensively and consulted on evidence-based nursing practice internationally. Dr. Luquire has been named an outstanding alumna from both TWU and UT.

Margaret L. McClure, EdD, RN, FAAN

Margaret McClure is a professor at New York University, where she holds appointments in both the School of Medicine and the College of Nursing. For almost 20 years she was the Chief Nursing Officer at NYU Medical Center, where she also served as the Chief Operating Officer and Hospital Administrator. She is currently involved in several national projects, most notably the American Academy of Nursing's Workforce Commission. As a part of that work, she co-chairs the Committee on the Educational Preparation of the Workforce.

A prolific writer and lecturer, Dr. McClure is internationally recognized as a nursing leader. Her best-known contribution to the literature is *Magnet Hospitals: Attraction and Retention of Professional Nurses*, which she co-authored under the auspices of the American Academy of Nursing. In 2002, she completed a new volume, *Magnet Hospitals Revisited*, a compilation of all the work that has been done to date regarding this subject.

A graduate of the Lankenau Hospital School of Nursing in Philadelphia, Dr. McClure received her baccalaureate degree from Moravian College in Bethlehem, PA, and her master's and doctoral degrees from Teachers College, Columbia University.

Dr. McClure is a member of Sigma Theta Tau and a past president of the American Academy of Nursing and the American Organization of Nurse Executives. She is the recipient of numerous awards, including an honorary Doctor of Humane Letters degree from Seton Hall University and an honorary Doctor of Laws degree from Moravian College. She retired from the United States Army Reserves with the rank of Colonel.

Janice W. Moran, MPA, RN

Janice Moran is currently serving as the Assistant Director of Operations for the Magnet Recognition Program for the American Nurses Credentialing Center. She comes to ANCC after 28 years of serving in the United States Navy Nurse Corps, retiring as a Captain. She has been with ANCC for the last eight years, serving in various position of the Magnet Recognition Program. Prior to coming to the ANCC, Moran was the Chief Nursing Officer at the National Naval Medical Center, Bethesda, MD.

Shirley H. Morgan, MSN, RN, NEA-BC

Shirley H. Morgan is currently serving as the Assistant Director for Development for the Magnet Recognition Program at the American Nurses Credentialing Center. A nurse executive for over 20 years, Ms. Morgan served as the Chief Nurse Executive at Prince George's Hospital Center in Cheverly, MD, a reputational magnet. Her experience includes teaching at the undergraduate levels at the University of Alabama at Birmingham, Georgia State University in Atlanta, GA, and Tuskegee University, Tuskegee, AL. A Johnson and Johnson Wharton Fellow in executive leadership and recipient of the Maryland Nurse's Association Pathfinder Award, she is a member of the American Organization of Nurse Executives.

Cecelia Mulvey, PhD, RN

Cecilia Mulvey is a Professor Emeritus at Syracuse University, where she served as Associate Dean for Academic Affairs and Interim Dean of the College of Nursing. Dr. Mulvey served as President of the American Nurses Credentialing Center from 2000 to 2005. A prolific lecturer, Dr. Mulvey is internationally recognized as a nursing leader. Throughout her career, Dr. Mulvey has advocated for the advancement of nurses and the nursing profession through credentialing.

Patricia Reid-Ponte, DNSc, RN,NEA-BC, FAAN

Patricia Reid-Ponte is currently serving as the Senior Vice President, Nursing and Patient Care Services, Dana-Farber Cancer Institute, and the Director, Oncology Nursing and Clinical Services at the Brigham and Women's Hospital in Boston Massachusetts. She is the Chair-Elect of the Commission on Magnet and has been a commissioner representing the American Academy of Nursing since 2006. Dr. Reid-Ponte is well known for her work with patient safety and was the co-principal investigator on a Commonwealth Fund and National Patient Safety Foundation study exploring the role of patients and clinicians as safety advocates. She received her bachelor's degree in nursing from the University of Massachusetts, Amherst, and her master's and doctorate degrees from Boston University. Dr. Reid-Ponte completed a three-year Robert Wood Johnson Nurse Executive Fellowship in 2004 and is a fellow of the American Academy of Nursing.

Margaret Elizabeth Strong, MSN, RN, NE-BC

Margaret Elizabeth Strong is an assistant professor in nursing at the Baptist College of Health Sciences. Mrs. Strong was a nurse executive for 25 years prior to becoming an educator. She has been a Magnet Commissioner for the past seven years representing long-term care. Mrs. Strong is a member of Sigma Theta Tau and has served in leadership positions in the Tennessee Nurses Association and the Tennessee Center for Nursing. She has received numerous state and local leadership awards.

Pamela Klauer Triolo, PhD, RN, FAAN

Pamela Klauer Triolo received her Bachelor of Science in Nursing from the College of St. Teresa, Winona, MN, and a Master's of Science in Nursing from St. Louis University, St. Louis, MO, with a major in Maternal-Newborn Nursing and Certification in Nurse Midwifery. Dr. Triolo earned a Doctor of Philosophy in Health Sciences Education, Instructional Design, and Technology from the University of Iowa, Iowa City, IA. Dr. Triolo's extensive clinical background is in critical care and women's health.

Dr. Triolo has held numerous leadership roles in both service and academe. Formal positions have included Chief Nursing Executive and Senior Vice President, The Methodist Hospital in Houston, TX; Associate Dean and Chief Nursing Officer, University of Nebraska Medical Center; a number of leadership positions at the University of Iowa Hospitals and Clinics; and the Director of Nursing Strategy and Innovation for the University of Texas M.D. Anderson Cancer Center in Houston, TX.

Dr. Triolo was also the Chief Nursing Officer for the University of Pittsburgh Medical Center (UPMC), which included 20 hospitals and 40,000 employees with over 11,000 RNs in Western Pennsylvania and internationally. She held a dual appointment as the Associate Dean for Academic-Service Partnerships with the University of Pittsburgh School of Nursing.

She is a consultant and author, and President, Principled Leadership Solutions, Houston, TX. She is also a fellow of the American Academy of Nursing.

Gail A. Wolf, PhD, RN, FAAN

Gail Wolf is currently a Clinical Professor at the University of Pittsburgh School of Nursing, where she is responsible for the master and doctoral programs in Nursing Leadership. Prior to this appointment Dr. Wolf spent 23 years at the University of Pittsburgh Health Care System in a variety of leadership roles, including ten years as the Chief Nursing Officer for the system. Dr. Wolf is currently the Chairperson of the Commission on Magnet and has served on the Commission on Magnet representing academe and the Academy of Nursing since 2001.

Dr. Wolf received her Baccalaureate in Nursing from West Virginia University, her master's in Nursing from the University of Kentucky, and her doctorate in Nursing Administration and Organizational Psychology from Indiana University in Indianapolis, IN. She is a Wharton Fellow and has served as President of the American Organization of Nurse Executives. She has published and lectured extensively throughout the United States, Australia, Italy, Japan, Canada, and Finland on issues relating to leadership of patient care.

Deborah Zimmermann, DNP, RN, NEA-BC

Deborah Zimmermann is the Chief Nursing Officer and Associate Dean at Virginia Commonwealth University Health System in Richmond, VA. For over 20 years she was a nurse executive in Rochester, NY. While in New York, she served as President of the New York Organization of Nurse Executives, and facilitated the introduction of legislation raising the educational requirements for New York State Registered Nurses. Dr. Zimmermann has worked with the Deans of New York State Colleges, the New York State Legislature, the New York State Board of Nursing, and healthcare leaders on a comprehensive plan to advance the profession to better meet the needs of the population since 2006. As a member of the Commission, she participated in the redesign of the national standards for Magnet designation, which were instituted in October 2009.

Magnet®: The Next Generation—Nurses Making the Difference

The First Generation

Margaret L. McClure, EdD, RN, FAAN

It requires a very unusual mind to undertake the analysis of the obvious.
Alfred North Whitehead, English philosopher and mathematician

In essence, science is a perpetual search for an intelligent and integrated comprehension of the world we live in.
Cornelius Bernardus Van Neil, U.S. microbiologist

The Magnet Hospital movement has become an amazing force for improving patient care across the United States and, indeed, around the world. While interest in this endeavor has been gaining momentum in recent years, the program's origins actually date back to the late 1970s, a time when our nation was experiencing a very serious nursing shortage. Not only was the shortage disturbing in those years because of its deleterious effect on patient care, it was also of concern because this workforce problem seemed to be cyclical in nature, recurring every few years, and rooted in issues that never were permanently resolved.

In response to this 1970s shortage, the country's major nursing organizations mounted a variety of tried and true efforts to address the shortage. At the time, the American Academy of Nursing (AAN) was a relatively new national organization, inaugurated in 1973 to serve the profession as a "think tank." Formally, its mission is to generate, synthesize, and disseminate nursing knowledge in such a way as to make pertinent data and research findings available to inform health policy. Thus, the membership comprises leaders who have the ability to influence not only nursing, but also the larger society.

AAN appointed the Task Force on Nursing Practice in Hospitals, charged to develop ideas for tackling this thorny shortage problem plaguing the nation's hospitals. Four AAN fellows were asked to serve. I was privileged to be appointed chair, and even more privileged to have three other knowledgeable and creative fellows totally committed to the work at hand.[1]

From the start, we knew we needed to attack the crux of the problem—the retention of professional nurses in hospitals. Most inpatient facilities were experiencing high turnover rates. They were able to attract new nurses, but were unable to keep them for substantial lengths of time.

During our first meeting, Mabel Wandelt described an earlier study she had conducted on nurse turnover in Texas hospitals. One observation became key to our work: during her data collection, she would often find herself in a city with one hospital that was not experiencing difficulty in attracting and retaining RNs. In fact, sometimes those institutions had waiting lists for nurses seeking positions.

The Task Force quickly realized that the literature was replete with opinion articles, and a handful of studies, regarding the causes of RN turnover, but there was no comparable research on the factors leading to retention. On further review, it became evident that the two variables— remaining versus resigning—were not opposite sides of the same coin. Individual nurses might well have very different motives for quitting versus continuing to work in their places of employment.

Further exploration of the literature confirmed our impressions. The lack of data regarding the fundamental requirements for a satisfying workplace environment for employees in general, and nurses in particular, was absent from the human resources knowledge base. It was at this point that the task force decided to conduct a nationwide study to identify those variables necessary to attract and retain professional nurses in hospitals.

It is worthwhile to note two circumstances. First, AAN had never conducted any research before; this, therefore, was a new direction for the organization. As a result, there was a great deal of discussion, and even some controversy, since funding the project was problematic. It is certainly a credit to those serving on the board that they were such risk takers, willing to make a substantial investment in the Task Force's proposed work.

Second, at the time the Task Force began its research, Thomas J. Peters and Robert H. Waterman—both well-known consultants and faculty members at the Stanford Business School—were hard at work on a similar study. Their book, *In Search of Excellence: Lessons from America's Best-Run Companies*, became one of the all-time best sellers in the management literature. Peters and Waterman (1982) addressed the factors that made organizations successful, including components related to employee job satisfaction. This widely read volume not only made millions of dollars for the authors, it also became the basis for many exemplary innovations that continue today among the world's leading corporations.

---

1 Members of the task force: Muriel A. Poulin, EdD, RN, FAAN, professor/chairperson, in Nursing Administration, Boston University; Margaret D. Sovie, PhD, RN, FAAN, associate dean for nursing practice, University of Rochester; Mabel A. Wandelt, PhD, RN, FAAN, professor and director, Center for Healthcare Research, University of Texas at Austin.

THE MAGNET HOSPITAL STUDY

The Sample

Without question, one of the first challenges was identifying a sample of successful hospitals. Using a Bureau of Labor Statistics model as our guide, we divided the United States into eight geographic regions. We then asked AAN fellows in each region to nominate from six to ten hospitals that had good reputations for recruiting and retaining nurses, using the following criteria:

- Nurses considered the hospital a good place to work.
- The hospital had a relatively low turnover rate.
- The hospital had competition for staff from other hospitals and agencies.

To ensure a valid sample we chose AAN nominators who were not employed by any hospital.

Originally, we thought there would be overlap among the hospitals nominated in each region, and this would help us choose the participants. Not so! In fact, of the 165 institutions named, there were virtually no duplicates.

We decided to call these facilities "magnet hospitals" at the suggestion of task force member Margaret Sovie. She noted that some schools in Rochester, NY, were called "magnet schools" and this would be an entirely appropriate label, since the organizations involved attract and retain staff.

Once we had selected our Magnet hospitals, we sent the chief nursing officers (CNOs) a letter informing them of the study and asking them to participate. We included an extensive form for them to submit, in which they described their institution, various staff characteristics, and their RN turnover rates.

As we awaited return of the CNOs' data forms, the task force conducted a pilot study in one region. We did so using only the descriptions submitted by the nominators. To our disappointment, it was immediately apparent that several of the institutions chosen were not, in fact, Magnet hospitals. Interviews with staff nurses were totally revealing in this regard. As a consequence, we refined our sampling procedures to make RN turnover rates the true defining factor for inclusion in the study. That single variable separated the Magnets from the non-Magnets.

From the 165 hospitals nominated, 46 qualified for the sample and 41 were able to participate in the study. Interestingly, they represented a diverse cross sample with varying characteristics, including:

- Size: 99 to more than 1,000 beds
- Occupancy: 72% to 98%
- Ownership: private (not-for-profit); private (for-profit); and governmental
- Non-union and unionized staffs

The sample, then, was fairly representative of our nation's hospitals.

Data Collection

A central location was chosen in each region for data collection, which was accomplished using in-depth interviews. Each hospital was represented by its CNO and a staff nurse, specifically someone assigned to direct patient care and non-managerial duties on a daily basis. The CNOs were interviewed in the morning; the staff nurses later in the day. We did this to assure staff nurses that their confidentiality would not be breached.

For both groups, the interviews consisted of the same nine, open-ended questions starting with, "What is it about your hospital that makes it a good place for nurses to work?" The remaining questions were essentially probes on the first, to better understand the specific factors that might be important in creating a positive environment. For example, we explored the involvement of staff in hospital programs and committees, nurse–physician relationships, nurse–supervisor relationships, and the image of nursing within the institution.

The Findings

Our study findings have been extensively reported elsewhere. (McClure et al., 1983; McClure & Hinshaw, 2002). They can best be summarized as the following 14 characteristics:

Quality of nursing leadership: Nursing leaders were perceived as knowledgeable and strong risk takers who followed an articulated philosophy in the day-to-day operations of their nursing departments. They also conveyed a strong sense of advocacy for, and support of, the staff.

Organizational structure: The structures of the hospitals were described as being decentralized, with active nursing representation evident on organizational committees, councils, etc. In addition, the CNO served at the executive level of the organization and, in almost every case, reported directly to the chief executive officer (CEO).

Management style: Across the institution, administrators practiced a participatory style of management, incorporating staff opinions and input into their decision-making. In particular, the nurse executives were viewed as visible and accessible, encouraging open communication through a variety of means. These individuals were not strangers to their staffs.

Personnel policies and programs: Salaries and benefits were reported to be generally competitive with and occasionally ahead of others in their communities. Work schedules proved to be especially important, with every effort made to involve the staff in the creation of flexible staffing models, with a minimum of required shift rotation. The nurses indicated that this careful attention to their hours reflected respect from their employers, and was highly valued.

Professional models of care: Magnet hospitals were noted for their adoption of models of care that gave nurses both the responsibility and the authority for the provision of care to their patients. Nurses were viewed as true professionals, expected to be accountable for their practice, and the coordinators of the total care their patients received.

Autonomy: The models of care served to imbue the nurses with a sense of autonomy that was reflected in their concern for standard setting and monitoring of care, at both the unit and organization levels.

Quality of care: Clearly, the nurses in the study perceived that they were providing very high-quality care to their patients. Moreover, they believed that the entire organization was committed to standards of excellence, and gave credit to their nursing leaders for actively creating an environment where such practice was valued.

Quality improvement: In keeping with the pursuit of high-quality patient care, there was evidence of efforts underway to continually assess and improve care delivery throughout the organization. It should be noted that the idea of "quality assurance" was in its infancy in those years. Therefore, it was interesting that the nurses in this study understood they were on the cutting edge and were proud that their organizations were adopting such processes. Moreover, they welcomed their own participation in these activities.

Consultation and resources: There were numerous specialized clinical resources available to both nurses and physicians, and the staff nurse participants viewed this as particularly helpful to care delivery. Among those singled out for comment were a variety of clinical nurse specialists, some of whom were in managerial roles.

Community and the healthcare organization: The hospitals in the study had a strong community presence, and nurses were very involved in a variety of outreach programs. These proved rewarding as they developed networks to help meet clinical and educational needs for patients and colleagues across the continuum of care.

Image of nursing: The image of nursing in the hospitals was considered very positive. In virtually every instance, participants said that nursing was viewed as competent and credible, resulting in their feeling valued and respected. This positive image prevailed among administrators, patients, the community, and, most important, the nurses themselves. What appeared especially significant was the fact that the nurses felt supported by nursing and hospital administrators, whom they credited with creating an environment in which interdisciplinary collaboration was encouraged and even expected.

Professional development: The hospitals placed a strong emphasis on personal and professional growth and staff development. The focus on in-service, and continuing and formal education, was viewed as contributing to the improvement of patient care and was especially important to the nurses in the study. In particular, they valued opportunities for competency-based clinical advancement, including clinical ladders.

Teaching: One of the most prominent findings was the high value nurses—particularly staff nurses—placed on education and teaching. Not only were they interested in education for their own personal and professional growth, they valued their role as teacher of others. Very positive attitudes were also apparent in relation to students and affiliated educational programs.

Interdisciplinary relationships: Interdisciplinary effort and shared decision-making were perceived as essential ingredients. A sense of mutual respect was exhibited among all disciplines.

The study was published as a monograph in 1983 under the title *Magnet Hospitals: Attraction and Retention of Professional Nurses* (McClure et al., 1983). And while the nursing community expressed great enthusiasm, others within the healthcare industry were not as positive. This was chiefly because the shortage had begun to abate. As a result, it was no longer a high priority for hospital administrators, trustees, and others.

Lessons Learned

The task force did not conduct any further research. However, we did maintain informal contact with many subjects from our study. These interactions provided a wealth of additional information regarding the climate and the positive features of magnetism.

First and foremost is the lesson that most institutions, even the best of today's Magnet-designated hospitals, do not yet fully comprehend. Simply stated, Magnet status is not purely a nursing designation. While it is true that nurses lead the program and nursing departments are the driving forces behind it, Magnet achievement is not possible without the participation and support of the entire organization. The hospital either embodies the necessary exemplary corporate culture or it does not. It is either a place in which all employees find satisfaction in their work or it is not. It is impossible for hospitals to provide a rich and rewarding environment for nurses alone. Every individual—from the CEO to the entry-level employee—affects, and is affected by, the quality of the workplace environment.

That said, the fact that nurses are the driving force behind Magnet should come as no surprise. Nursing is a hospital's core business. Patients are admitted to inpatient facilities because they need nursing care, and they are discharged when their needs can be met in another environment. And while nurses deliver a great deal of the care themselves, they also have the responsibility to pull together the contributions of the other departments and disciplines that serve their patients. In this regard, they are often called *coordinators* of care. However, I prefer a more meaningful term: *integrators* of care. Integration means the nurse at the bedside ensures that patient needs are met in a timely, competent, and safe manner. This involves engaging with a wide range of staff members from physicians to housekeepers, from pharmacists to security officers. No one is unimportant to patient care and therefore to the work of the nurse. As a result, the Magnet designation is an institutional award—one that should make everyone in the organization proud.

We learned a second lesson early on: Magnet recognition brings valuable business benefits. Our study wasn't even published before one of the CNOs told an interesting story. Her CEO asked her to meet with a group that was determining the bond rating for their hospital. He specifically asked her to describe the Magnet hospital study and the reasons their institution was included in the sample. As a result of that meeting, the hospital received a very favorable upgrade in its bond rating. This turned out to be the first of a number of similar stories that have continued to this day.

The third lesson we learned is that a Magnet environment can be transitory. It requires constant attention and cultivation to flourish. A number of the early Magnet hospitals lost their ability to attract and retain staff over time, while others became increasingly successful in doing so. Many factors contribute to the persistence or demise of such a workplace climate. However, two stand out as particularly important: 1) a change in the CEO, and 2) a change in the CNO. This lesson speaks loudly to the role of executive leadership and its impact on the overall organization. Having learned from it, the American Nurses Credentialing Center (ANCC) wisely determined that Magnet designation would be temporary. Hospitals that achieve it must regularly undergo the same rigorous review.

FURTHER RESEARCH

While the original subjects' anecdotes were useful and helpful, the Task Force was keenly aware that very few major changes are ever made as a result of one small study. Fortunately, several of nursing's most able scientists were intrigued by our work and set out to do further research on the same hospitals. Building on the original foundation, these scholars added incrementally to our knowledge of the variables involved in the creation of rewarding clinical practice settings. Their findings served to both replicate the original research and provide vital new insights to guide hospital management.

The first to undertake such work was Marlene Kramer. Her initial study sought to determine the extent to which Magnet hospitals demonstrated the same characteristics as the corporations that Peters and Waterman (1982) studied for their groundbreaking research . Not surprisingly, her findings were positive and she went on to conduct many other studies, using first the original Magnet hospitals and later the ANCC-designated Magnet hospitals (Kramer & Schmalenberg, 1988a, 1988b).

Most important, these later studies uncovered the evidence that Magnet hospitals create positive outcomes, not just for their staff, but also for their patients. Of particular significance was the first study conducted by Linda H. Aiken and her colleagues at the University of Pennsylvania. They set out to investigate whether Magnet hospitals had lower Medicare mortality rates than comparable non-Magnet hospitals (Aiken et al., 1994). They found that the mortality rate was significantly lower in Magnet hospitals, a result that highlighted the likely impact of the nursing practice environment on critical patient outcomes.

Aiken's group went on to conduct a number of other studies, comparing Magnet with non-Magnet hospitals in relation to such important subjects as the mortality rate of AIDS patients, the cost of nurse staffing, and job satisfaction and nurse-assessed quality (Aiken, 2002).

Because of this impressive and growing body of evidence, the American Nurses Association charged the ANCC to develop a formal program that would identify and reward special status to those institutions that were achieving excellence in patient care through positive practice environments. In 1994, ANCC launched its Magnet Recognition Program® and formally designated its first Magnet hospital, the University of Washington Medical Center in Seattle.

The 14 characteristics in the original study findings became the foundation for all that followed. As you will read in the ensuing chapters, the Magnet Recognition Program has evolved and grown based on the continuous accumulation of knowledge during the several decades that Magnet hospitals have existed.

The original Magnet hospital study represented a true beginning of evidence-based practice in hospital and nursing administration. More important, ANCC's Magnet Recognition Program has continued to serve the entire healthcare industry, setting the gold standard for clinical management practices that many emulate, including institutions not seeking Magnet designation. These standards have changed over time, and will continue to do so, as evidence from the field is collected and assessed. In every case, the true beneficiaries are the hospital staff members and the patients they serve.

REFERENCES

Aiken, L. H., Smith, H. & Lake, E. T. (1994). Lower Medicare mortality among a set of hospitals known for good nursing care. *Medical Care, 32*(8), 771–787.

Aiken, L. (2002). Superior outcomes for Magnet hospitals: The evidence base. In M. McClure & A. Hinshaw (Eds.). *Magnet hospitals revisited: Attraction and retention of professional nurses.* Washington, DC: American Nurses Publishing.

Kramer, M., & Schmalenberg, C. (1988a). Magnet hospitals: Institutions of excellence. Part I. *Journal of Nursing Administration, 18*(1), 13–24.

Kramer, M., & Schmalenberg, C. (1988b). Magnet hospitals: Institutions of excellence. Part II. *Journal of Nursing Administration, 18*(2), 11–19.

McClure, M., & Hinshaw, A. (Eds.). (2002). *Magnet hospitals revisited: Attraction and retention of professional nurses.* Washington, DC: American Nurses Publishing.

McClure, M., Poulin, M., Sovie, M., & Wandelt, M. (Eds.). (1983). *Magnet hospitals: Attraction and retention of professional nurses.* Kansas City, MO: American Nurses Association.

Peters, T. J., & Waterman, R. H. (1982). *In search of excellence: Lessons from America's best-run companies.* New York, NY: Harper and Row.

2

Establishing the Recognition Program

Jeanne Floyd, PhD, RN, CAE
Cecilia Mulvey, PhD, RN

It is my personal conviction and testimony that the "magnet movement" in all its manifestations
and nuances offers the greatest hope for the future of nursing and healthcare organizations.
Margretta Madden Styles in McClure and Hinshaw (EDs.), *Magnet Hospitals Revisited*, 2002, p. xii

Throughout history, nurses have led the way in creating environments and conditions
conducive to patient healing. As the creator of modern nursing, Florence Nightingale observed
the deplorable conditions in the military hospital at Scutari and accepted the challenge to
reform nursing care. Her vision brought order to the environment and resulted in a cultural
transformation, promoting healing and markedly reducing mortality. Following in the
Nightingale tradition, the Magnet journey transforms the hospital culture and environment to
support the best nursing care possible.

The Magnet Recognition Program® is integral to the portfolio of credentialing programs
and services offered by the American Nurses Credentialing Center (ANCC), which was
incorporated as a subsidiary of the American Nurses Association (ANA) in 1991. The term
"credentialing" is used in both the national and international language of nursing and was
popularized following the publication of the ANA *Study of Credentialing in Nursing: A New
Approach* (ANA, 1979) and *Specialization and Credentialing in Nursing Revisited* (Styles et al.,
2008). Credentialing includes efforts to describe the provision of quality care (ANA, 1979;
Urden & Monarch, 2002, p. 103).

LAUNCHING THE PROGRAM

Interestingly, development of the Magnet Recognition Program has been intertwined with the development and evolution of ANCC. The "birthing process" began in 1987 when the ANA Board of Directors appointed a Consultant Advisory Panel for Accreditation of Nursing Services. This was in response to the Magnet hospitals study, published by the American Academy of Nursing in 1983, which identified 41 facilities across the country that successfully attracted and retained—like a magnet—professional nursing staff in a time of shortages. The study found that these hospitals had re-designed the work environment to include:

- A practice setting with congruence of values at all levels of the organization.
- A clear vision and actualization of the roles of the professional nurse.
- Consistent administrative support regarding the value of staff and patients.

The ANA panel recommended development of a program to recognize excellence across a broad spectrum of nursing services, including care delivered in the community and long-term care facilities. As a first step, ANA leadership approved development of standards for organizational nursing services and responsibilities for nurse administrators across all settings. Additional strategic discussions followed, and in 1990 the ANA board approved a feasibility study to create a national program to recognize excellence in nursing services. This was to be a collaborative, evidence-based effort, in partnership with key nursing organizations, and founded on application of ANA standards. The ANA Congress on Nursing Practice and Economics and the Council on Nursing Administration commissioned the study.

Study results led the ANA Board of Directors to approve establishment of a national recognition program for organized nursing services within ANCC. The program would provide recognition to healthcare facilities that excelled in creating work environments that imbedded the philosophy, practices, and leadership to support exemplary nursing practice and quality patient care. Because recruitment and retention of nurses were of paramount concern nationwide, staff nurse involvement was a foundational element and has become a unique cornerstone of the program over time.

In addition, ANA invited members of the Council on Nurse Executives (an ANA interest group) to evaluate ways to motivate excellence in nursing practice. Council chair Mary S. Tilbury, EdD, RN, NEA-BC, recalls considerable discussion around translating the Magnet hospital findings into "a program that would allow every organization to aspire to those characteristics and attributes" (Margaret McClure in Houser & Player, 2007, p. 213).

In its first report to the ANA board in 1991, the ANCC board requested approval of the establishment of a national recognition program to serve as a "magnet" for organized nursing services. The credential conferred would recognize institutions for promoting an organizational culture that rewarded professional practice excellence. The ANA board approved the program and named Marie Reed, EdD, RN, NEA-BC, the first director of ANCC.

Concurrent with program development activities, Marlene Kramer, MSN, RN, and Claudia Schmalenberg, PhD, RN, FAAN, began a multifaceted study of Magnet-recognized hospitals that greatly expanded the understanding of what staff nurses identified as important to nursing effectiveness. The research began in 1984 and continued through 2001. It identified the following essentials of magnetism:

- Working with other nurses who are clinically competent
- Good nurse–physician relationships and communication

- Nurse autonomy and accountability
- A supportive nurse manager or supervisor
- Control over nursing practice and practice environment
- Support for education (in-service, continuing education, etc.)
- Adequate nurse staffing
- Concern for the patient paramount (Kramer & Schmalenberg, 2002)

These seminal research findings captured the staff nurse perspective and increased understanding of the components that led to the Forces of Magnetism. The results influenced the Magnet Recognition Program's early development and continue to have an impact.

In 1991, Frances Harpine, PhD, RN, was named Magnet project director for the next phase of development of the Magnet Recognition Program. Dr. Harpine was a tenured professor at Catholic University School of Nursing, where she taught research processes and design. She also served as a site visitor for the National League for Nursing. An Internal Steering Committee/External Advisory Board guided program development. Members included:
- ANA Board member Claire Murray;
- ANCC Board member Thomas Stenvig;
- ANA Congress of Nursing Practice representative Linda Sawyer;
- ANA Congress of Nursing Economics representative Helen Ripple;
- Former chair of the Council on Nursing Administration Mary Tilbury; and
- Constituent Assembly Executive Committee representative Maureen Shekleton.

The Committee guided development of the National Magnet Recognition Program for Excellence in Nursing Service and outlined program components.

In 1993, Dr. Harpine left her position and Dr. Tilbury was invited to further develop the Magnet program. There was no budget, so she worked Saturdays for six months. With the help of an administrative assistant, she developed manuals for appraisers and applicants, created bylaws for the Commission on Magnet Recognition (COM), and planned a pilot study. These were all steps along the way to developing a credentialing process for organizations that were to be recognized for excellence in nursing services. The original 41 Magnet hospitals, now called "reputational Magnets," were offered the opportunity to reaffirm their status in the new program before other organizations applied for Magnet status. Not one of them had any interest in participating in the formal program. Since they had not yet obtained a credential, ANCC required them to stop using the term "Magnet designation." They could say they were among the original 41 studied in the research, but they could not advertise that they were Magnet unless formally designated under the new criteria (Margaret McClure in Houser & Player, 2007, p. 213).

Dr. Tilbury designed a pilot study that used a random stratified sampling technique based on the five bed-size categories identified by the American Hospital Association. Four states were selected: Washington, New Mexico, Alabama, and Massachusetts—one from each time zone. Three waves of invitations were sent to hospitals falling into each bed-size sampling cell by sampled state. Once an invitation was accepted, the cell was closed in that state. Some cells were never filled. The pilot study revealed that hospitals with 300 or more beds were the primary market (Margaret McClure in Houser & Player, 2007, p. 215).

During the time when the program was being developed, appraisers were selected. The nurses in this elite group were the first peer reviewers who were educated and prepared to review hospital nursing services in applicant hospitals. The 12 original Magnet appraisers were:
- Phyllis Ethridge, MS, RN, NEA-BC, FAAN (Arizona);
- Helen Hoesing, PhD, RN, NEA-BC, FACHE (Nebraska);
- Frances T. Feldsine, MSN, RN, NEA-BC (New York);
- E. Carol Polifroni, EdD, RN (Connecticut);
- Dorothea Milbrandt, MS, RN (Michigan);
- Catherine E. Neuman, MSN, RN, NEA-BC (Illinois);
- Jeanette S. Matrone, PhD, RN (Rhode Island);
- Joan M. Caley, MS, RN, CS, NEA-BC (Washington);
- Larry Hepner, MSN, RN (Maryland);
- Anne Scott, MSN, RN, CS, NE-BC (Virginia);
- Sheila P. Englebardt, PhD, RN, NEA-BC (North Carolina); and
- Anne Jones, MS, RN (Minnesota).

The University of Washington Medical Center was the first Magnet-recognized organization in the pilot study. In 1994, ANCC and Magnet staff believed the program was ready to launch and publicly announced that applications were welcome. Although ANCC's budget did not carry a line item for the program, it made a commitment to hire a dedicated, full-time staff member. Dr. Tilbury, as Magnet project consultant, assumed the responsibility of part-time director, spending at least one day a week in the ANCC office (Margaret McClure in Houser & Player, p. 214).

Hackensack University Medical Center in New Jersey was the first applicant facility under the official Magnet program. Chief Nursing Officer (CNO) Antoinette (Toni) Fiore, MA, RN, had observed the 41 hospitals in the original study and followed the progress of the Magnet pilot program. She appointed Stephanie Goldberg, MSN, RN, as the Hackensack Magnet project coordinator, and the team developed its application based on the proposed Magnet criteria and outcomes of an organizational gap analysis. Goldberg recalled that the purpose of the Magnet journey at Hackensack was to integrate a successful work environment, not to collect an award. Magnet standards became the Hackensack operational framework long before the application was submitted (Margaret McClure in Houser & Player, p. 219).

Many would acknowledge that Hackensack was the first to put the Magnet program on the map. After it achieved Magnet status, the medical center conducted a significant multimedia advertising campaign that educated the public on how designation set the bar for patient care excellence (Margaret McClure in Houser & Player, p. 219).

Magnet program components revolved around indicators of a quality nursing service, including elements such as organizational structure, nursing leadership, professional development opportunities, and control over nursing practice. Nursing staff turnover rates, retention and longevity, agency nurse support, and efficient utilization of personnel through staff mix ratios also were considered. A variety of education and practice indicators were identified. Examples included application of professional standards to guide the nursing department practices, investment in the continued development of nursing staff, appropriate employment of advanced practice nurses, and placement of nursing specialists in an environment requiring their knowledge, skills, and abilities.

Meanwhile, ANCC was organizing the credential for Magnet designation. The COM was the body that bestowed the credential on organizations that met the standards of excellence. The COM held its first meeting in 1995. The executive committee comprised:
- Chairperson Peggy K. Jones, MSN, MBA, RN, NEA-BC;
- Vice Chairperson Sheila Englebardt, PhD, RN, NEA-BC; and
- members at large Jacqueline A. Dienemann, PhD, RN, FAAN and COM members:
  - Elizabeth M. Egleston, BSN, RN;
  - Marjorie Peck, PhD, MSN, RN;
  - Donna Kulawiak, BA;
  - Claire Mailhot, EdD, RN, FAAN;
  - Elizabeth M. Newton, MSN, RN;
  - Maureen E. Shekleton, DNSc, FAAN;
  - Jean Welch, MS, RN, C, NE-BC; and
  - Margaret L. McClure, EdD, RN, FAAN.

In 1996, the COM was named in the ANCC bylaws. Chairperson Peggy Jones joined the ANCC board as an ex-officio, non-voting member. Within a few months, the COM added a long-term care representative and renamed the program Magnet Nursing Services Recognition. That same year, a labor complaint surfaced in a Magnet hospital in the mid-Atlantic. The ANA board put the Magnet program on hold while an inquiry was conducted to ensure that the hospital with the labor complaint met all the core criteria and standards. The COM conducted its own investigation to ensure that the Magnet program's criteria and standards adequately addressed the issues relevant to the current delivery of nursing services. In the end, the COM upheld the decision to grant the hospital Magnet status and the program resumed.

Such an in-depth programmatic review ultimately strengthened the Magnet program. Application instructions were revised to require the following:
- Organizations approved for site visits must post a 30-day invitation for public comment.
- Organizations must place appraisal documents in a public area such as the library, where employees and the public can examine them.
- Organizations must notify and invite comment from ANA, constituent member state nurses associations, and other interested parties.

Responses would be integrated into the review process and an appellate body identified to hear final appeals, if necessary.

The Magnet program continued to grow in other ways, especially in the linkages to safety and quality. On behalf of the COM, Sheila M. McCarthy, MSN, RN, and Margaret D. Sovie PhD, RN, FAAN, wrote the white paper "Quality Indicator Report," which discussed ways to integrate quality indicators into the application process (McCarthy & Sovie, 1977). The indicators incorporated performance improvement elements from the Joint Commission and the ANA Nursing Care Report Card for Acute Care. McCarthy and Sovie posited that the program needed to include balanced measurement of structure, process, and outcome indicators. They recommended that institutions seeking Magnet recognition have the opportunity to measure nurse-sensitive indicators such as pressure ulcers, nosocomial infection rates, and patient fall rates along with quality management and performance improvement. Patient satisfaction measurement held a pivotal place in the provision of quality care. In their enlightened thinking, McCarthy and Sovie believed that future advancements in the science of measurement and clinical information systems would foster agreement in identification of second-generation indicators such as those found today in the National Database of Nursing Quality Indicators® (NDNQI®).

In 1998, the Magnet program was expanded to include long-term care facilities. Identified services included sub-acute, chronic, rehabilitation, psychiatric, and other emerging care of vulnerable populations. However, only one long-term care facility was ever recognized, and re-designation did not follow. Currently, ANCC's new Pathway to Excellence® Program appears better suited to meet the needs of the long-term care community. This program recognizes and credentials organizations that demonstrate and describe the elements of a positive working environment for nurses.

In 2002, Magnet Nursing Services Recognition was renamed the Magnet Recognition Program for the purpose of recognizing excellence in four major areas:
• Management, philosophy, and practice of nursing services;
• Adherence to national standards for improving the quality of patient care;
• Support for professional practice and continued competence of nurses; and
• Understanding and respecting the cultural and ethnic diversity of patients, their significant others, and healthcare providers.

By this time, international interest in the program was growing. The change in title occurred, in part, as a result of observations among the international community that patient care issues are rarely the focus of a single healthcare provider discipline. Rather, care is associated with interdisciplinary contributions and efforts. International colleagues pointed out that while nursing is a significant focus of the Magnet program, nurses do not care for patients in isolation. Successful patient outcomes are the result of care from a team.

STRENGTHENING THE MAGNET RECOGNITION PROGRAM

The Magnet Recognition Program is continually reviewed and evaluated. As evidence accumulates, processes are carefully adjusted to improve program validity. In 2002, when it became apparent that the program needed an appeals policy, a document was developed that addressed the requirements across the credentialing programs. This was to ensure that each organization received fair consideration of expressed concerns. The COM would review only the material used in making the initial credentialing decision and the appeals-related material submitted by the appellant. In 2003, stakeholder feedback led to changes in eligibility, practice, and documentation requirements for Magnet aspirants. The review process became more intense, raising the bar both for initial applicants and re-designating organizations.

Later, the COM worked closely with consultant Pamela Triolo, PhD, RN, FAAN, to increase the rigor of the program. Dr. Triolo made 25 recommendations that were implemented from 2005 to 2007:
• Part I called for a redesign of the Magnet appraiser application. Careful scrutiny was given to appraiser qualifications and the selection process. Chief executive officers (CEOs), CNOs, and academic deans would identify new appraisers. It was essential that team leaders have experience as CNOs in Magnet-recognized facilities.

- Part II addressed the Magnet appraiser team constellation, and led to the development of Magnet mentors and Magnet fellows. Documented evidence showed that as the size of the Magnet appraisal team increased, inter-rater reliability was enhanced. Another bonus: larger teams also meant shorter site visits.
- In Part III, the need for differentiated appraiser training was identified. Seasoned appraisers were provided quarterly webinar updates, and each took Gallup's Strengths Finders Index 2.0 (Rath, 2007). This gave staff useful information to organize strong appraisal teams. Magnet fellows received in-depth training and were assigned Magnet mentors.
- Part IV adjusted appraiser compensation.
- In Part V, the appraisal process was re-engineered to reflect increased efficiency and transparency. Until this time, appraisal of blinded documents was the norm. This was changed to unblinded reviews in keeping with processes followed in other recognition programs. The number of COM members was increased.
- Parts VI and VII centered on technological upgrades to the database in the Magnet program office for applications and Commission decisions. This new database was nicknamed "Maggie" in honor of original Magnet researcher Margaret McClure. The Maggie database eventually gave appraisers web-based access and the ability to document site visits results via the Internet.

Triolo's document ended with the recommendation that the "Future of Magnet" be considered in the next evolutionary wave of refinements to the Magnet criteria. This eventually led to the development of the new Magnet Model and Vision, introduced in 2008 (*See* The Magnet Vision).

The new Magnet Model provides a fresh perspective on the Sources of Evidence and how they interplay to create a work environment that supports excellence in nursing practice. Using a combination of factor analysis, cluster analysis, and multidimensional scaling, final Source of Evidence scores were examined to determine how they might be organized based solely on their empirical properties. The results suggested an alternative framework for grouping the Sources of Evidence, collapsing them into fewer domains than the 14 FOM. The empirical model yielded from the analysis informed the conceptual development of the new Magnet Model. Evidence-based practice, innovation, evolving technology, and patient partnerships are evident (*See* Figure 2-1). The Magnet Model includes an overarching theme of global issues in nursing and health care. To provide greater clarity and direction, as well as eliminate redundancy, the new, simpler model organizes the 14 FOM into five components. It reflects a stronger focus on measuring outcomes and allows for more streamlined documentation, while retaining the 14 FOM as foundational to the program. The COM created a new vision to communicate the importance of Magnet organizations in shaping future changes that are essential to the continued development of the nursing profession and to quality outcomes in patient care (*See* The History of the Magnet Recognition Program).

> **The Magnet Vision**
> Magnet organizations will serve as the fount of knowledge and expertise for the delivery of nursing care globally. They will be solidly grounded in core Magnet principles, flexible, and constantly striving for discovery and innovation. They will lead the reformation of health care; the discipline of nursing; and care of the patient, family, and community.
> *Commission on Magnet Recognition, 2008*
> Source: ANCC, 2008

Figure 2-1. The Magnet Model

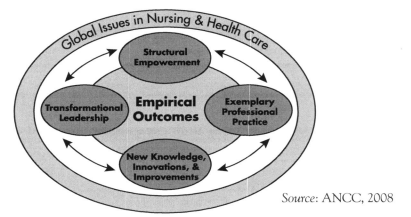

Source: ANCC, 2008

The History of the Magnet Recognition Program (Urden & Monarch, 2002)

1983—The American Academy of Nursing's (AAN) Task Force on Nursing Practice in Hospitals conducted a study of 165 hospitals to identify and describe variables that created an environment that attracted and retained well-qualified nurses who promoted quality patient/resident/client care. Forty-one of the 165 institutions were described as "magnet" hospitals because of their ability to attract and retain professional nurses. The characteristics that seem to distinguish these organizations from others became known as the Forces of Magnetism (FOM).

1990—June. Based on a recommendation of the ANA, the ANCC was established as a separately incorporated, nonprofit subsidiary through which ANA offers credentialing programs and services.
December. The initial proposal for the Magnet Hospital Recognition Program for Excellence in Nursing Services was approved by the ANA Board of Directors. The proposal indicated that the program would build on the AAN 1983 Magnet hospital study.

1994—After completing a pilot project that included five facilities, ANCC designated the University of Washington Medical Center in Seattle as the first Magnet organization in the United States.

1997—ANCC changed the name to the Magnet Nursing Services Recognition Program. In addition, program criteria were revised using *Scope and Standards for Nurse Administrators* (ANA, 1996).

1998—The Magnet Nursing Services Recognition Program was expanded to recognize nursing excellence in long-term care facilities.

2000—In response to requests, the program was expanded to recognize healthcare organizations abroad.

2002—The name was changed to the Magnet Recognition Program®.

2007—ANCC commissioned a statistical analysis of Magnet appraisal team scores from evaluations conducted using the 2005 *Magnet Recognition Program Application Manual.* This analysis clustered the Magnet criteria (Sources of Evidence) into more than 30 groups which yielded an empirical model for the Magnet Recognition Program.

2008—With input from a broad representation of stakeholders, COM developed a conceptual model for Magnet and a vision for the future. The five-component model integrates the 14 FOM.

Magnet Recognition Program Directors	**Magnet Recognition Program Commission Chairs**
Jennifer Matthews, PhD, APRN-BC	Peggy K. Jones, MSN, MBA, RN, NEA-BC
1997–1999	*1995–1997*
Kammie Monarch, MSN, RN, JD	Sheila P. Englebardt, PhD, RN, NEA-BC
2001–2004	*1997–2001*
Elaine Scherer, MA, BSN, RN	Linda D. Urden, DNSc, RN, CNS, NE-BC, FAAN
2004–2007	*2001–2005*
Karen Drenkard, PhD, RN, NEA-BC, FAAN	Brenda J. Kelly, MA, RN, NEA-BC
2008–present	*2005–2009*
	Gail A. Wolf, PhD, RN, FAAN
	2009–2010
	Patricia Reid-Ponte, DNSc, RN, NEA-BC, FAAN
	2010–2012

The program was further strengthened in 2008 when Karen Drenkard, PhD, RN, NEA-BC, FAAN, became director. Under her guidance, improvements continued including appraiser training with post-testing to ensure appraiser competency. On-site training addressed customer service and behavioral expectations of appraisers during site visits. Additionally, the waiting list for Magnet application scheduling was eliminated. Staff and customer satisfaction surveys registered an all-time high satisfaction level. (*See* Magnet Recognition Program Directors and Commission Chairs.) To date, 377 hospitals have achieved Magnet status. These hospitals average 475 beds, have resources allocated to nursing services, have a higher percentage of BSN-prepared nurses, and are able to support the resources needed to meet the standards for Magnet recognition.

GROWTH OF THE DOMESTIC PROGRAM

To date, the Magnet Recognition Program has undergone geometric growth. The bars in Figure 2-2 represent the number of Magnet designations and re-designations from 1993 to 2010 year-to-date.

Figure 2-2. Magnet Designations and Redesignations

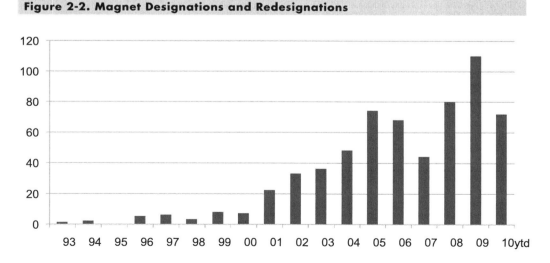

Year of Recognition

Source: ANCC, 2010

History of the Magnet Conference

1997 Charter Magnet Conference, Atlanta, GA
- Sponsored by Saint Joseph's Hospital, Atlanta
- 200 participants
- Keynote JoEllen Koerner, MS, RN, FAAN: "The Keys to Improving Nurse Satisfaction"
- Linda Aiken, PhD, RN, FAAN: "Quality Outcomes in Magnet Hospitals."
- Diane Soules, University of Washington Medical Center: "Magnet Experience: Excellence in Nursing"
- Mary Ann Donohue, PhD, RN, Hackensack University Medical Center: "Magnet Experience: Understanding the Application Process"
- Kim Sharkey, MBA, RN: "Benchmarking: Comparing Best Practices"
- Jennifer Matthews, PhD, RN, CS: "Accreditation and the Magnet Recognition Program"

1998 Magnet Conference: Celebrate Nursing, Magnet Recognition: Achieving Excellence in Hospital Based Nursing Services
- Sponsored by Saint Joseph's Hospital, Atlanta, GA
- Speaker ANA President Beverly Malone, PhD, RN
- Speaker ANCC President Margretta Madden Styles, PhD, RN

1999 Magnet Conference
- Saint Joseph's Hospital, Atlanta, GA, invited ANCC to co-sponsor conference at Hackensack University Hospital

2000 Magnet Conference
- Hosted by University of Washington

2001 Magnet Conference
- Hosted by North Carolina Baptist Hospital, Wake Forest University Baptist Medical Center

2002 Magnet Conference
- Hosted by Mayo Clinic, Rochester, MN

2003 Magnet Conference
- Houston-based conference included M. D. Anderson Cancer Center as the lead facility, along with St. Luke's Episcopal Hospital and The Methodist Hospital

2004 Magnet Conference
- Collaborative conference with UC Davis, California Medical Center in Sacramento

2005 Magnet Conference
- Miami conference canceled because of Hurricane Katrina

2006 Magnet Conferences
- To compensate for the 2005 conference, two conferences were held in 2006
- Spring 2006: Baptist Hospital of Miami, South Miami Hospital, Miami Children's Hospital and Holy Cross Hospital collaborated to hold an event in Miami
- Fall 2006: Denver, CO led by University of Colorado Hospital, The Children's Hospital, Craig Hospital, and Poudre Valley Hospital

2007 Magnet Conference
- Atlanta, GA
- Co-hosts included Saint Joseph's Hospital as lead sponsor, Medical Center of Central Georgia, St. Joseph's/Candler, and the University Hospital of Augusta

2008 Magnet Conference
- Salt Lake City, UT
- Intermountain Health Care as sponsor with other Utah Magnet hospitals

2009 Magnet Conference
- Louisville, KY
- Over 5,000 attendees
- Five Magnet Hospital partners for sponsorship:
  —Baptist Hospital East
  —Kosair Children's Hospital
  —Central Baptist Hospital
  —St. Elizabeth Healthcare
  —University of Kentucky Hospital

2010 Magnet Conference
- Phoenix, AZ
- Magnet Hospital sponsors include:
  —Banner Good Samaritan Medical Center
  —John C. Lincoln North Mountain Hospital
  —Scottsdale Healthcare – Shea/Osborn
  —University Medical Center Tuscon

The program focuses on three goals:
- The promotion of quality in a setting that supports professional practice;
- The identification of excellence in the delivery of nursing services to patients and residents; and
- The dissemination of "best practices" in nursing services.

ACHIEVING ACCREDITATION FOR THE MAGNET RECOGNITION PROGRAM

ANCC is the largest global nurse credentialing center, so it stands to reason that as leaders and staff spoke with potential international clients, the topic of program accreditation would surface. The discussion would go something like this: "ANCC and the Magnet Recognition Program essentially accredit or recognize the structures, processes, and outcomes of healthcare organizations. Who accredits the Magnet program?" Dr. Styles was an early proponent of International Standards Organization (ISO) accreditation for Magnet. But after she left the ANCC presidency, the notion was largely forgotten. In 2005, as international interest in ANCC's programs and services continued to grow, the executive director, Dr. Jeanne Floyd, presented the ANCC board with a plan to seek ISO accreditation (also known as certification) for the entire organization. The Magnet Recognition Program and the Accreditation Program achieved ISO 9001:2000 accreditation in 2007. The credential indicates that the recipient:
- Has a system in place to deliver consistent services;
- Conducts periodic internal audits to ensure that its key processes are functioning as intended; and
- Has a system for preventive and corrective action with an eye toward improving the overall management system. (Personal communication, MaryMoon Allison, Director of Quality Management Systems, ANCC).

NATIONAL MAGNET CONFERENCE

Magnet's key philosophical underpinning is the mentoring and sharing of new knowledge development, practice innovations, and lessons learned. Saint Joseph's of Atlanta achieved Magnet recognition in 1995 and sponsored the charter Magnet conference two years later. Approximately 200 nurses participated.

Today the annual National Magnet Conference has grown to over 6,000 participants, with nurses attending from around the world. The conference brings together all levels of nurses to celebrate and advance the work of nursing. Features include the Art of Magnet Nursing Gallery and the Magnet Film Festival where bedside nurses tell their stories. The visionary nurses of Saint Joseph's of Atlanta deserve our gratitude for initiating the Magnet Conference, which has become a core gathering place for all Magnet nurses. Fifteen years ago this group of pathfinders could not have imagined how much joy and celebration the conference would generate among nurses. This is the sole nursing conference that transcends hierarchical positions and clinical silos, and brings together vertical teams of chief nurses, nurse managers, and bedside clinicians in a celebration and advancement of nursing practice. The Magnet Conference supports camaraderie, generosity of spirit, and professional partnership that promotes sharing and advancement of nursing practice across all boundaries. (*See* History of the Magnet Conference.)

BUILDING A MAGNET COMMUNITY

In keeping with the Magnet philosophy of sharing and support, ANCC is building learning communities that offer nurses in Magnet facilities opportunities to interact with and learn from one another. The idea was born at the 2001 Magnet Conference. Magnet CNOs met with ANCC president Cecilia Mulvey and executive director Jeanne Floyd and affirmed the importance of communication and connection as in any community. The first generation of connection and community was through an electronic community. CNOs are now connected through a listserv, where they "meet" electronically to discuss policies, procedures, successful practices, and problems. Within moments of posting, helpful responses begin to appear. The community has expanded to include Magnet program directors and research directors. Like the CNOs, they meet at the annual conference and remain connected on the listservs during the year.

Sharing and connection are important to the international nurse community, too. Requests for ANCC's international study tours increase every year. Nurses from around the world want to learn more about credentialing programs, and Magnet recognition in particular. The study tours include a day with Magnet staff and CNOs from local Magnet facilities, followed by visits to several Magnet-recognized hospitals.

The Magnet community truly entered the global arena when Sigma Theta Tau International and ANCC collaborated to use the Virginia Henderson International Library as the electronic repository to post abstracts selected for presentation at the National Magnet Conference. Magnet facilities also may post research abstracts and practice innovations that might benefit global colleagues. The repository is available around the clock, free of charge.

ANCC debuted its online learning communities in 2010 and continues to perfect them. Each learning community represents a component of the new Magnet Model: Transformational Leadership; Structural Empowerment; Exemplary Professional Practice; and New Knowledge, Innovations, and Improvements. They offer Magnet hospitals and those on the Magnet journey a formal mechanism to engage with experts in evidence-based practice, research, quality outcomes, innovations, and exemplary practice environments. As well, the intent is to create innovative ways of sponsoring domestic and international research. Each learning community includes exemplars from actual Magnet applications that illustrate best practices. Feedback from the pilot program indicates that the communities help disseminate new knowledge at a rapid rate, showcase good work and innovation, and are groundbreaking and powerful in their capacity to form new learning circles composed of novice and expert nurses.

ANCC's Institute for Credentialing Research is sponsoring an initiative to facilitate multi-site clinical nursing research. ANCC's Research Council is conducting the pilot study, which unites approximately 42 Magnet hospitals to examine outcomes in congestive heart failure patients. The study will yield not only clinical results, but also lessons learned in how to manage research

Magnet Prize Recipients

- 2003: The Patient Safety Center team at the James A. Haley Veterans Hospital in Tampa for its seminal research in patient and staff safety.
- 2004: The University of Colorado Medical Center for its evidence-based practice to improve clinical and management outcomes.
- 2005: The Mayo Clinic for its Nursing Genomics Program.
- 2006: The American Academy of Nursing for its transformational research, *Magnet Hospitals: Attraction and Retention of Professional Nurses.*
- 2007: Pitt County Memorial Hospital in North Carolina for creating the Bariatric Consortium that addressed issues related to morbidly obese patients.
- 2008: Abington Memorial Hospital in Pennsylvania for its innovative Daily CARE Plan, which actively involves patients in care decisions.
- 2009: Colorado's Poudre Valley Hospital for its community case management.

with large databases and the factors that support generalized findings. Additional future studies should evolve, further uniting the Magnet community to conduct research that improves patient outcomes across all regions of the country and perhaps around the world.

THE MAGNET PRIZE

The COM first endorsed the idea of a Magnet Prize in 1991, and Dr. Cecilia Mulvey created the actual prize 12 years later. The prize rewards exemplary innovation in Magnet-recognized facilities. Those who apply must demonstrate how they have "raised the bar" in their hospitals and improved patient outcomes.

Few applied at first, but the number of applications has gradually increased. It is evident that each institution has examined its practices and developed exemplary innovations that add to the body of nursing knowledge, thereby transforming the practice of nursing. Each recipient has spoken at the National Magnet Conference, inspiring others to pursue advancements in their hospitals. Currently, the prize carries a purse of $25,000, provided by the Cerner Corporation and ANCC (*See* Magnet Prize Recipients).

THE MAGNET MOVEMENT

Margretta Madden Styles's vision for nursing—that the "Magnet movement" offers the greatest hope for the future of nursing and healthcare organizations—continues to be realized. In less than two decades, Magnet recognition is fulfilling a promise to transform the image and reality of professional nursing practice. Today's nurse leaders, from the executive to the staff nurse, are contributing to the movement's momentum. New graduates seek initial positions in Magnet-recognized facilities, and experienced nurses hone and sharpen their practice to ever-increasing levels of excellence.

The original study (McClure et al., 1983) posed two main questions:
- What are the important variables in the hospital organization and its nursing service that create a magnetism that attracts and retains professional nurses on its staff?
- What particular combination of variables produces model(s) of hospital nursing practice in which nurses receive professional and personal satisfaction to the degree that recruitment and retention of qualified staff are achieved?

Around the globe nurses have responded to the call inherent in these two questions and developed innovative strategies to transform the links between nursing care and patient outcomes. The developing Magnet community strives to use the Magnet journey as a foundation for discovery and continual improvement.

What does the future hold for the next generation of nurses? The Magnet Recognition Program and the research and evidence-based Sources of Evidence provide every new nurse with the framework and standards that are essential to a positive practice environment. The Magnet standards need to be in place in every healthcare organization, as the evidence is building that the linkages between a positive practice environment for the healthcare workers leads to positive quality outcomes for the patients. Thanks to the research of those who came before us we know the answers to many of these questions about creating a positive practice environment for nurses and other healthcare workers for the ultimate achievement of excellence in outcomes. The nurses who care for their patients are grateful to the researchers who set the bar at a high level of excellence.

REFERENCES

American Nurses Association. (1979). *Study of credentialing in nursing: A new approach.* Washington, DC: Author.

American Nurses Association. (1996). *Scope and standards of nurse administrators.* Washington, DC: Author.

American Nurses Credentialing Center. (2008). *Application manual: Magnet Recognition Program.* Silver Spring, MD: Author.

Houser, B. P., & Player, K. N. (2007). *Pivotal moments in nursing: Leaders who changed the path of a profession* Vol. 2. (Chapter, "Margaret L. McClure", pp.168–223). Indianapolis, IN: Sigma Theta Tau International.

Kramer, M., & Schmalenberg, C. (2002). Staff nurses identify essentials of magnetism. In M. L. McClure & A. S. Hinshaw (Eds.), *Magnet hospitals revisited: Attraction and retention of professional nurses.* Washington, DC: American Nurses Publishing.

McCarthy, S., & Sovie, M. (1977) Quality Indicator Report. (January 25). Unpublished internal document. Silver Spring, MD: American Nurses Credentialing Center.

McClure, M. L., & Hinshaw, A. S. (Eds.). (2002). *Magnet hospitals revisited: Attraction and retention of professional nurses.* Washington, DC: American Nurses Publishing.

McClure, M. L., Poulin, M., Sovie, M., & Wandelt, M. (1983). *Magnet hospitals: Attraction and retention of professional nurses.* Kansas City, MO: American Nurses Association.

Rath, T. (2007). *Strengths finder 2.0.* New York, NY: Gallup Press.

Styles, M. M., Schumann, M. J., Bickford, C. J., & White, K. (2008). *Specialization and credentialing in nursing revisited: Understanding the issues, advancing the profession.* Silver Spring, MD: American Nurses Publishing.

Urden, L. D., & Monarch, K. (2002). The ANCC Magnet Recognition Program: Converting research findings into action. In M. L. McClure & A. S. Hinshaw (Eds.), *Magnet hospitals revisited: Attraction and retention of professional nurses.* Washington, DC: American Nurses Publishing.

3

The Next Generation

Gail Wolf, PhD, RN, FAAN
Pamela Triolo, PhD, RN, FAAN
Patricia Reid-Ponte, DNSc, RN, NEA-BC, FAAN
Karen Drenkard, PhD, RN, NEA-BC, FAAN
Janice Moran, MPA, BSN, RN

Reprinted with permission from *Journal of Nursing Administration*
Vol. 38, Number 4, pp. 200–204
© 2008 Wolters Kluwer Health/Lippincott Williams & Wilkins

Do not go where the path may lead, go instead where there is no path and leave a trail.
Ralph Waldo Emerson

Twenty-five years ago, the foundation of the Magnet Recognition Program® was established. Magnet® designation has served as the hallmark of excellence for nursing practice, and research has demonstrated a profound impact on nursing practice and patient care. The purpose of this article was to forecast the direction of the Magnet Recognition Program and describe the transition to a more outcomes-focused model. The authors discussed the results of a multivariate structural analysis of the Forces of Magnetism and the subsequent future model for Magnet.

Magnet designation is the highest level of recognition that the American Nurses Credentialing Center can accord to healthcare organizations that provide the services of registered professional nurses. For 25 years, the term *Magnet hospital* has been equated with excellence in nursing and patient care. Although it has been widely acclaimed, the Commission on Magnet

(COM) felt it imperative to continually refine and improve the Magnet program to keep pace with today's challenging healthcare environment.

In 1981, the American Academy of Nursing established a Task Force to study the organizational factors distinguishing a small number of hospitals that had been unusually successful in maintaining competent nurse workforces during a time of serious nursing shortages. The Task Force identified 41 hospitals that served as "magnets" for professional nurses; they were able to attract and retain a staff of well-qualified nurses and were therefore consistently able to provide quality care (McClure et al., 1983). This vanguard group of hospitals served as the "reputational Magnets" and were the precursors of the current Magnet Recognition Program. An analysis of these hospitals' characteristics revealed 14 consistent components that became widely known as the Forces of Magnetism (FOM). Magnet status is not a prize or an award. It is a credential that recognizes nursing excellence. In the early 1990s the American Nurses Association implemented a Magnet Recognition Program housed in the subsidiary organization, the American Nurses Credentialing Center, and based on the original study. As part of the credentialing process, the Commission on Magnet was appointed to oversee the program. In 1998, the program was expanded to include long-term care facilities, and in 2000, it was extended again to accommodate applications from international healthcare organizations.

THE MAGNET PROGRAM TODAY

As the outcomes demonstrated by Magnet facilities have became more widely known both publicly and professionally, the demand for Magnet designation has grown. There are currently 377 Magnet-designated facilities. Applications for Magnet designation have grown at an average of 32% per year for the past five years.

Maintaining a program this successful requires the collaboration of many stakeholders. Magnet-designated organizational leaders have identified additional ways in which the program could be improved, and as the number of Magnet-accredited organizations has grown, additional data have afforded an even greater opportunity for analysis and refinement.

In 2004, COM launched the first comprehensive evaluation of the Magnet Recognition Program since the 1990s. In 2005, the commission approved 25 recommendations for changes to the Magnet program (Triolo et al., 2006). These recommendations included clarifying the characteristics and developmental needs of successful appraisers, including the composition of teams; shifting the review process from blind to transparent; balancing the scoring of the FOM among process, structure, and outcome; and creating a dynamic model for the FOM, as well as other recommendations designed to increase the efficiency of the appraisal process. Implementation of these recommendations has created extensive paradigm shifts in the program designed to support program excellence. The work continues today.

THE NEXT GENERATION MAGNET PROGRAM

Building on the recommendations unanimously approved by the Commission in March 2005, the Commission began to work on a new model for the FOM that would bring greater clarity to how the forces worked in a systematic way to reinforce and result in excellence in nursing practice. Although the 14 forces had served the program well, the goal was to reduce redundancy and move to a dynamic model to illustrate contemporary research on organizational behavior. A multivariate analysis of the 14 FOM and the Sources of Evidence was possible now that a sufficient number of facilities were Magnet-designated. Two to four appraisers rated 147 Magnet facilities on 164 Sources of Evidence. Data were subjected to factor analysis, cluster analysis, and multidimensional scaling. The analysis revealed the 14 FOM carried a fair amount of redundancy and could be measured by seven domains or "clusters" of evidence: leadership, resource utilization and development, nursing model, safe and ethical practice, autonomous practice, research, and quality processes.

Understanding that the 14 FOM could be measured by seven domains of evidence was a break-through finding. The COM felt that if changes to the standards and streamlined requirements were implemented, it would eliminate a great deal of redundancy, provide greater focus for organizations, and simplify the application process. However, this analysis only focused on the existing Magnet program or "where we have been." It did not answer the question "Where do we need to go?" The Commission needed a conceptual model to guide the future development of Magnet principles for the highest performance in healthcare organizations.

NEXT STEPS: VISION TO REALITY

Although the Magnet program has served the nursing profession and health care well for the past 20 years, there is evidence to suggest that health care is going through a major reformation. Changes in patient populations, providers, technology, and medicine demand new models of care. Factors such as patient partnerships, evidence-based practice, new technology, and innovation are key to our success in the future (Wolf & Greenhouse, 2007).

Magnet organizations are poised to be the pioneers and innovators of future best practice. However, in a desire to maintain Magnet accreditation, many Magnet hospitals seek stability in order to achieve re-designation. The COM determined that a different standard for evaluating initial versus redesignating organizations was needed to facilitate this transformation.

The original Magnet Recognition Program was primarily focused on structure and processes within an organization and contained only one FOM dedicated to quality outcomes. Although structure and process are important, the true measurement of organizational success rests in its outcomes. The COM felt that it was critical to create an eighth domain for Magnet dedicated to this concept. This domain, focusing on results, is common in other models, in particular the Baldrige model. Commissioners considered that although structure and process were important for excellence, the outcomes of the infrastructure were essential to a culture of excellence and innovation.

THE VISION FOR MAGNET

In 2007, the COM adopted a new vision statement for the Magnet Program (ANCC, 2008):

> Magnet organizations will serve as the fount of knowledge and expertise for the delivery of nursing care globally. They will be solidly grounded in core Magnet principles, flexible, and constantly striving for discovery and innovation. They will lead the reformation of health care; the discipline of nursing; and care of the patient, family, and community.

In addition, the COM wanted to develop a new model for Magnet that would incorporate the eight new domains and provide a "roadmap" for the Magnet journey. To do so, an invitational summit was held in the summer of 2007. Thirty experts from across the country came together to review the new domains of Magnet, examine Sources of Evidence that supported these domains, and explore various models that could be used.

THE MODEL FOR MAGNET

The new Magnet Model, based on expert review and adopted by the Commission, is shown in Figure 3-1.

The Magnet Model is composed of five components: Transformational Leadership; Structural Empowerment; Exemplary Professional Practice; New Knowledge, Innovations, and Improvements—all of which lead to the component, Empirical Outcomes. Overarching the model are global issues in nursing and health care that acknowledge the various factors and challenges facing nursing and health care today. The following describes each of the Magnet components, the domains they contain, and weighting for both the initial designation and re-designation of Magnet organizations.

Figure 3-1. The Magnet Model

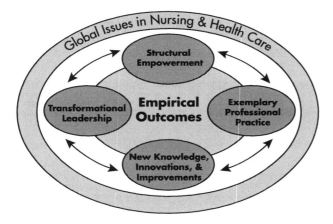

Source: ANCC, 2008

Transformational Leadership

Today's healthcare environment is experiencing unprecedented and intense reformation. Unlike yesterday's leadership requirement for stabilization and growth, today's leaders are required to transform their organization's values, beliefs, processes, and behaviors. It is relatively easy to lead people where they want to go; the transformational leaders must lead people where they need to be to meet the demands of the future. This requires vision, influence, clinical knowledge, and expertise in professional nursing practice and leadership. It also acknowledges that transformation may create turbulence and involve innovative approaches to solutions.

The organization's senior leadership team creates the vision for the future and the systems and environment necessary to achieve that vision. The organization's senior leaders must enlighten the organization as to why change is necessary and their part in achieving that change. They must listen, challenge, influence, and affirm as the organization makes its way into the future. Gradually, this transformational way of thinking should take root in the organization and become even stronger as other leaders adopt this way of thinking.

Within this concept, we find the original Magnet Forces of quality of nursing leadership and management style. They are measured by the new domain called Transformational Leadership. The intent is no longer just to solve problems, fix broken systems, and empower staff, but to actually transform organizations to meet the future. Magnet organizations today strive for stabilization; however, healthcare reformation calls for a type of controlled destabilization that gives birth to new ideas and innovations. This leadership is essential for initiating the Magnet journey, and therefore, this concept is weighted more heavily on initial designation than on re-designation based on the belief that leadership that is truly transformational will become hardwired into the organization and visible through the outcomes that the organization is able to achieve.

Structural Empowerment

The structure of an organization is designed to operationalize the mission, vision, and values and achieve the necessary outcomes. This begins with leadership and is accomplished through the organizational strategic plan, structure, systems, policies, and programs. Staff needs to be developed, directed, and empowered to accomplish the organizational goals and achieve desired outcomes. This may be accomplished through a variety of structures and programs: clearly, one size does not fit all.

The original Magnet forces of professional development, image of nursing, nurses in the community, organizational structure, and policies and programs are contained within this concept and measured by the domain of resource utilization and development. This concept is weighted more heavily upon initial designation; once the structure has been established and hardwired into place, good outcomes should result.

Exemplary Professional Nursing Practice

The true essence of a Magnet organization stems from exemplary professional nursing practice. This entails a comprehensive understanding of the independent and dependent role of nursing. It includes the application of that role with patients, families, communities, and the interdisciplinary team and the application of new knowledge and evidence.

The original forces of Magnet contained within this concept include models of care, autonomy, interdisciplinary relations, resources and consultation, and nurses as teachers. They are measured by four of the new domains: models that guide practice, safe and ethical practice, autonomous practice, and quality processes. Within this concept, we need to incorporate future requirements of professional practice, such as patient and family partnerships, interdisciplinary collaboration, workforce and patient safety, the impact of technology, and continuity of care.

For an organization seeking Magnet status, this area of professional practice initially needs a great deal of attention. However, the goal is more than the establishment of strong professional practice, it is what that professional practice can subsequently achieve. As a Magnet organization matures, the outcomes of professional practice deserve more merit, and thus, this concept is weighted more heavily on redesignation.

New Knowledge, Innovations, and Improvements

Strong leadership, the right structure, and exemplary practice are essential building blocks for Magnet organizations but are not the final goal. Magnet organizations have an ethical and professional responsibility to contribute to patient care, the organization, and the profession in terms of new knowledge, innovations, and improvements. Our current systems and practices need to be constantly evolving, redesigned, and redefined if we are to be successful in the future.

This concept embraces the original Magnet force of quality improvement, measured by the new domain of research. However, this concept is intended to move beyond a basic application of research to include evidence of redesign, new models of care, application of new evidence to guide practice, and visible contributions to the science of nursing.

It is difficult for an organization to develop new knowledge, innovations, and improvements until it is well established and grounded in Magnet principles. Organizations that are in the re-designation cycle should have the reinforcing structure and processes in place, and the focus should be on outcomes that are tracked, trended, and improved over time, as well as benchmarked against other high-performing organizations. Thus this concept is weighted more heavily on re-designation.

Empirical Quality Results

Today's Magnet designation process has a primary focus on structure or processes, with an assumption that good outcomes will follow. In the previous Magnet Model, outcomes were not specified and were minimally weighted. There were no quantitative outcome requirements for Magnet designation or re-designation. Until recently, we have lacked any type of benchmark data that would allow comparisons with best practice. This area is where the greatest change is evident in the new Magnet Model. With over 300 Magnet facilities, the data sources for comparison are now significant.

Having a strong structure and processes is only the first step. The question for the future is not "What do you do?" or "How do you do it?" but rather "What difference have you made?" Magnet organizations are in a unique position to become the pioneers and innovators of the future and demonstrate best-practice solutions to the numerous problems inherent in our healthcare systems today. They may do this in a variety of ways through innovative structure and various processes, and they must be recognized, not penalized, for their inventiveness.

This concept contains the Magnet force of quality of care but goes beyond that concept to look at outcomes. Outcomes are categorized into clinical outcomes related to nursing, workforce outcomes, patient and family outcomes, and organizational clinical outcomes. Outcome data that the organization routinely collects will be used based on quantitative benchmarks. These outcomes will form the basis of the "report card" of a Magnet organization, a way to graphically demonstrate excellence. These outcome data are used for the interim reports and provide a simple way of demonstrating that a Magnet organization remains on track.

The past Magnet designation process (2005) put relatively little weight on outcomes. In the new model (2008), weighting of outcomes exceeds that of structure and process, with more weighting applied to outcomes in re-designating hospitals. A summary of the new model concepts, the original 14 FOM, and the eight new domains can be seen in Table 3-1.

Table 3-1. Relationship of the Forces of Magnetism, Domains of Evidence, and Magnet Model Concepts

Forces of Magnetism	Domains of Evidence	Magnet Model
Nursing leadership Management style	Leadership	Transformational Leadership
Professional development; Image of nursing; Organizational structure; Personnel policies and programs; Community	Resource utilization and development	Structural Empowerment
Professional models of care; Autonomy; Interdisciplinary relations; Consultation and resources; Nurses as teachers; Quality of care: ethics, patient safety, and quality infrastructure; Quality improvement	Professional practice model; Safe and ethical practice; Quality processes; Autonomous practice	Exemplary Professional Nursing Practice
Quality improvement; Quality of care: research and evidence-based practice	Research	New Knowledge, Innovations, and Improvement
Quality care	Outcomes	Empirical Quality Results

Source: ANCC, 2008

IMPLEMENTATION OF THE NEW MAGNET PROGRAM

In the fall of 2007, the proposed changes to the Magnet program were presented at the Magnet annual conference. Additional input, suggestions, and evidence-based Sources of Evidence were solicited. Based on that input the 2008 *Application Manual* was finalized and became operational in the summer of 2008.

Appraisers are leading expert nurses who represent a range of professional expertise and experience-based knowledge. To familiarize Magnet appraisers with the 2008 manual a series of competency-based training sessions were conducted in 2009 to ensure equitable levels of reliability, clarity of the Magnet Sources of Evidence, and accuracy in the appraisal process.

CONCLUSION

For the past 25 years, Magnet designation has been equated with excellence. Health care is now poised for reformation, and what worked in the past will not necessarily work in the future. By adopting the proposed changes in the Magnet program, Magnet organizations will not only maintain excellence but also become the pioneers and innovators for the future of healthcare delivery and professional nursing practice. The stakes are high and the time is here. Nurses stand at the forefront of possibility to make the changes necessary to move us into a different future for health care. Transformational nursing leaders of Magnet hospitals are poised to lead the way to improve patient outcomes and improve the health of the communities we serve.

REFERENCES

American Nurses Credentialing Center. (2008). *Application manual: Magnet Recognition Program.* Silver Spring, MD: Author.

McClure, M. L., Poulin, M., Sovie, M., & Wandelt, M. (1983). *Magnet hospitals: Attraction and retention of professional nurses.* Kansas City, MO: American Nurses Association.

Triolo, P. K., Scherer, E. M., & Floyd, J. M. (2006). Evaluation of the Magnet recognition program. *Journal of Nursing Administration, 36*(1), 42-48.

Wolf, G., & Greenhouse, P. (2007). Blueprint for design: Creating models that direct change. *Journal of Nursing Administration, 37*(9), 381–387.

4

Transformational Leadership

Gail Wolf, PhD, RN, FAAN
Deborah Zimmermann, DNP, RN, NEA-BC
Karen Drenkard, RN, PhD, FAAN, NEA-BC

The very essence of leadership is that you have to have vision. It's got to be a vision you articulate clearly and forcefully on every occasion.
Theodore Hesburgh, President, Notre Dame University

A leader takes people where they want to go. A great leader takes people where they don't necessarily want to go, but ought to be.
Rosalyn Carter

The journey to Magnet® designation begins with Transformational Leadership. Unlike traditional leadership, Transformational Leadership changes organizational values, beliefs, and behaviors to achieve an optimal level of success. Transformational leaders have a clear picture of where the organization needs to be, and can successfully move followers to that place—even those initially reluctant to take the journey. Transformational leaders excel at creating a desired future state, which is the first step in forming a Magnet environment. Chief nursing officers (CNOs) in Magnet organizations work with their staff to develop a vision, articulate a model for professional practice, and oversee a strategic plan that provides the roadmap for success. Success happens not because followers dutifully agree to go along, but because leaders and followers learn from each other, come to common understanding, and establish shared values and beliefs. Thus, in a truly transformed organization, these values and beliefs live in the staff's DNA and drive their behavior.

None of this happens by accident. Becoming a transformational leader requires thoughtfulness, inclusivity, good listening skills, flexibility, and resiliency. Whether convincing others to create a healthy work environment or justifying the resources to become a Magnet facility, these qualities—plus a large dose of courage—are what transform vision into reality.

This chapter takes a closer look at the nuts and bolts of Transformational Leadership: its history, evolution, and importance in a developing Magnet facility. Exemplars from all levels— staff nurse, front-line manager, director, and CNO—illustrate how the Sources of Evidence for Transformational Leadership are actualized in Magnet hospitals.

HISTORY OF TRANSACTIONAL AND TRANSFORMATIONAL LEADERSHIP

James M. Burns was one of the first to introduce the concept of leadership in relation to both leader and follower. "The genius of leadership lies in the manner in which leaders see and act on their own and their followers' values and motivations," he wrote (Burns, 1978, p. 19). Transformational Leadership emerged from an understanding of transactional leadership, a relationship based on contingent rewards. In a transactional relationship, the leader provides resources and support in exchange for specific outcomes and employee behaviors. A salary and benefits, for example, are provided in return for completing work in a timely and responsible fashion. Burns defined transactional leadership as emphasis on work standards, assignments, task orientation, and task completion. The focus was on maintaining the status quo, with reward and punishment based on compliance.

While Burns proposed that leadership is both a transactional and a transformational process, it was Bass (1990), followed by other researchers (Avolio, Waldman & Yammarino, 1991), who identified the characteristics of Transformational Leadership:

- **Individualized consideration.** The ability of the leader to treat each person equally, but differently, to give personal attention; functioning as a coach or mentor (Atwater & Yammarino, 1993).
- **Intellectual stimulation.** The ability of the leader to ask questions and find ways to solve problems, to encourage followers to create solutions and try new ideas; questioning assumptions, reframing problems, approaching old situations in new ways (Avolio, Waldman & Yammarino, 1991).
- **Charisma.** The leader's ability to generate excitement and provide vision and a sense of direction.
- **Inspiration.** The leader's ability to communicate a shared vision to the follower; motivating and inspiring others by providing meaning and challenge to followers' tasks (Howell & Avolio, 1993).
- **Idealized influence.** The leader's ability to behave as a role model and emulate high ethical standards.

These characteristics translate easily into health care and nursing. Nursing leaders in Magnet organizations typically possess the characteristics described here and effectively use these attributes to achieve superior outcomes.

NURSING LITERATURE

Numerous studies in the nursing literature have explored and linked transformational nursing leadership to higher levels of nurse satisfaction, nurse retention, and work group effectiveness (Boyle, Bott, Woods, & Taunton, 1999; Dunham-Taylor, 2000; Dunham-Taylor & Klafehn, 1990; Failla & Stichler, 2008; Manojlovich & Laschinger, 2007). Transformational leaders foster healthy work environments that result in empowered nursing practice, fewer work-related injuries, greater use of evidence-based practice, and improved unit performance (Aarons, 2006; Bass, Avolio, Jung & Berson, 2003; Clarke, 2007). Nursing leaders who demonstrate certain identified behaviors create an environment where clinicians want to work effectively. While varied models and frameworks of leadership exist, the foundational work of core leadership attributes is evident in transformational leadership. The concepts of leadership theory as it impacts nursing practice have real implications for the delivery of health care. If a leader's characteristics, traits, and behaviors can impact the work environment, then these same characteristics, traits, and behaviors will influence the culture, the productivity, and ultimately the performance of an organization. The Sources of Evidence in Magnet's Transformational Leadership domain are based on the attributes identified in these studies and illustrated in Table 4-1.

CNOs in Magnet organizations tend to be highly transformational. It is evident in their ability to shape the environment, overcome obstacles, collaborate, communicate, and cultivate effective teams. They ensure that their clinical directors and managers possess the essential competencies and skills to create the preferred future. Then, with their teams, these nurse executives pursue well-defined goals with enthusiasm and passion. They focus on quality, purposeful work, a transparent journey, and a meaningful vision. Through their participative and integrative style, they help team members internalize the vision and make it their own.

ESTABLISHING A SHARED VISION

The first step is to work in a partnership of leaders and bedside clinicians to establish a vision that is meaningful to all clinicians and one that the entire nursing community is willing to work toward. A transformational leader sees beyond the organization's current state and creates a picture of a better future. This vision is measurable, achievable, and challenging. "We want to be the best we can be" is not a measurable vision. But "Achieving Magnet designation within three years" is measurable, achievable, and challenging. The leader then must demonstrate how commitment to this vision will meet everyone's interests.

Initially, the vision may seem overwhelming to followers. It is the transformational leader's role to offer a positive outlook and lead the way. The leader may not have all the answers, but knows how to tap the expertise of others to find them. The leader may encounter roadblocks, but has the flexibility to pursue opportunities and explore different paths. The leader may face setbacks, but has the courage to take risks. The leader may be challenged, but has the determination to remain focused on the vision.

With trust, authenticity, and honest communication, transformational leaders win over their followers who, in turn, continue the transformation. The voyage is difficult, and sometimes overwhelming, but old paradigms and values must change for the organization to achieve its full potential. Transformation is possible only when everyone is fully committed to the process.

Table 4-1. Transformational Leadership Characteristics

Leadership Characteristics Evident in Magnet Hospital Nurse Leaders[1]	Transformational Leadership Characteristics From the Research[2]
Change agent Charismatic Loyal Communicating effectively and openly Maintaining high standards and living up to expectations of staff Preserving a position of power and status within the hospital Infusing value into organization Including nurses in ethical issues management based on ANA's *Code of Ethics for Nurses*	*Idealized influence:* Charisma, respect, trust, confidence, ethics, and moral reasoning
Team building Visioning Visibility Active in state and national organizations	*Inspirational motivation:* Shared vision, direction, enthusiasm, team spirit, motivation
Continuing education and professional development emphasized Professional autonomy encouraged Critical thinking encouraged	*Intellectual stimulation:* Encourage followers to ask questions and find new ways to solve problems
Driving decision-making downward Actively involving staff in decision-making and goal setting Being supportive and knowledgeable Accessible and available for support, being responsive to staff needs Valuing each nurse's contribution to organization	*Individual consideration:* Encouraging followers to reach higher levels of potential and achievement

1 *Sources:* Armstrong, Laschinger, & Wong, 2008; Brady-Schwartz, 2005; Dunham-Taylor, 2000; Kramer & Schmalenberg, 1988; Laschinger & Finegan, 2005; Scott, Scholaski, & Aiken, 1999; Stordeur, Vandenberghe, & D'hoore, 2000; Upenieks, 2003. Column 1 reprinted with permission from M. Kramer and C. Schmalenberg, Magnet Hospitals: Part 1 & 2: Institutions of Excellence, *Journal of Nursing Administration*, 18(1), pp. 13-24, and 18(2), pp. 11-19. © 1988. Lippincott Williams & Wilkins. All rights reserved.

2 *Sources:* Bass et al., 2003; Burns, 1978; Chan & Drasgow, 2001; Chiok, 2001; Kouzes & Pusner, 1988. Column 2 reprinted with permission.

Here is how two organizations—at home and abroad—developed a vision, values, and strategic priorities for nursing.

> *Gladys Mouro is a true visionary leader. The CNO at the American University of Beirut Medical Center spearheaded a six-year journey to bring Magnet designation to the Middle East. Says Mouro: "I decided to embark on the Magnet journey the moment I recognized that it would raise the bar of quality to a level of excellence for our patients who deserve the very best." Applying for Magnet status in 2003 marked both the culmination of a long process to rebuild nursing services at the hospital after the 15-year Lebanese civil war and the beginning of an ambitious campaign to transform nursing practice and set nursing standards for the region. During the application process, Mouro and her colleagues introduced comprehensive improvements at the medical center. When the facility achieved Magnet status in 2009, Mouro told her staff, "We strive for the impossible and make it happen. That's what makes this place unique." (Mouro, 2009)*
>
> *In Rochester, NY, a new Chief Nursing Officer (CNO) faced the challenge of unifying staff from two organizations after a hospital in the health system closed. States their CNO: "Emotions were high, trust was low, and the vast majority of employees believed they had no control over their destiny. In a retreat with directors and chairs of a disenchanted self-governance council, the group openly and honestly discussed the organization's strengths, weaknesses, and desired future state. A staff nurse made a novel suggestion: why not pursue Magnet designation? The group deliberated, argued, and finally embraced the idea. The journey to Magnet became the vision, and the Forces of Magnetism provided the compass by which to guide decision-making over the next two years."*

In Rochester and Beirut, nursing leaders led the redesign of organizational policies and structures to create environments that promoted communication, innovation, and participation from those closest to the bedside. Clinicians were mentored to become experts in areas important to nurses, such as skin care, falls, anticoagulation, medication safety, and infection control. These unit-based staff experts then brought evidence-based practice to peers and new ideas from the bedside to larger hospital groups. In turn, staff experts set the priorities for organizational performance improvement.

Clinical nurses' role in decision-making is dependent on whether they are afforded time to participate in indirect clinical work. Without that guarantee from nursing leaders, teams cannot be held accountable for achieving measurable clinical outcomes. Potential solutions range from designating a day of the week or month for meetings to incorporating meetings into daily nurse assignments. Still, hurdles remain and ensuring consistent participation is a challenge in every organization. At one hospital, work away from the bedside was not perceived as "real work." Nurses felt they were neglecting their duties when they participated in planning sessions on a new electronic medical record, until the clinicians saw that new nurse-friendly protocols, developed by clinicians at the bedside, resulted in improved patient outcomes. It was at that point that all staff realized the impact of the work that was done by the clinicians who were temporarily away from the bedside. It reinforced to all staff that "real work" includes involvement in decision-making and promotes autonomy in practice. The support from senior nursing leaders to encourage participation in these assignments facilitated staff nurse autonomy.

The plan supporting an organization's Magnet vision and Magnet journey is comprehensive, detailed, and metric-driven. The vision becomes embraced by all staff and is a balance of being feasible—though many times a significant stretch from the current state—and flexible: all characteristics that Kotter has described as effective for driving transformational change (1996, p. 72).

It is vital that clinical nurses have open communication with nurse executives and other healthcare administrators. New ideas come from the edge, and in health care, that means those closest to patients. In the Magnet manual, the Sources of Evidence, or requirements, relating to visibility, accessibility, and communication are based on this premise. When staff nurses have a voice in the design of care standards, best practices are implemented and patient outcomes improve.

The CNO is responsible for creating an invigorating environment that promotes communication between nursing staff and hospital leaders. Frequent communication not only ensures adequate resources and personnel, but also creates a culture in which everyone takes equal responsibility for patient care. Good communication creates an environment of advocacy.

Sentara Health in Norfolk, VA, provides an example of good communication. Their CNO has introduced daily senior leader safety rounds. Every morning at 7:30 the chief executive officer, CNO, chief medical officer, and others review a daily report from the off-shift nursing supervisor, that prioritizes hospital rounding for that day. The leaders meet with staff, discuss issues, and, before the close of business, develop action plans. These daily communication rounds have resulted in improved staff morale and a reduction in patient falls. Walking rounds demonstrate how leaders in the organization value each nurse's contribution to the organization, and the results are tangible.

Open and frequent communication supports more effective advocacy for resources. At Advocate Christ Medical Center in Oak Lawn, IL, clinical staff nurses identified the need for an improved electronic medical record during regular unit nurse leader rounding. Because of the relationship of the nursing leaders with bedside nurses, the CNO was effective in advocating for the allocation of extensive resources for this effort. Staff from every specialty were then involved in the creation of a new computerized documentation system, which ensured its success.

Another demonstration of effective advocacy occurred at Memorial Hermann Memorial City Medical Center in Houston, TX. On behalf of staff, the CNO convinced the board of trustees to appropriate equipment and systems to implement a comprehensive program to improve flow and safety in the Emergency Department. The board approved more than $1 million to be spent on additional equipment and additional nursing staff as requested by the professional practice team—all necessary for a new split-flow care model, which in turn increased their ED volumes by 19% in just the first year. In addition it created an interdisciplinary communication system that significantly reduced turnaround time and enhanced patient flow.

LEADING TRANSFORMATION FROM ANY POSITION

Today's complex healthcare environment requires leadership at every level and from every position. This is possible in Magnet organizations because staff have access to resources and information that support patient care and professional growth. In a decentralized environment, nurse managers and bedside clinicians are positioned to exert significant influence on patient care processes and outcomes.

Establishing transformational leaders at every level of the organization is essential in achieving Magnet designation. When nurses are respected and valued members of the team, they are more likely to support a healthy work environment, which is key to patient safety (IOM, 2004). Nurses working in a supportive environment will actively promote wellness and remove safety threats. In fact, as is the case in the exemplar below, staff nurses in Magnet hospitals are often able to look beyond the boundaries of their own organization to improve the health and wellness of a community.

> *Transformational Leadership at the Bedside*
> *Nurses at First Health Moore Regional Hospital in Pinehurst, NC, proposed a community initiative to make their hospital campus smoke-free. This was no ordinary challenge: the hospital is located in the heart of tobacco country. Nurses advocated for this change in policy after a literature review indicated hospitalization facilitates long-term smoking cessation and a reduction in preventable cancers. After a year of community planning, countless smoking cessation classes, free nicotine replacement for employees, and implementation of a comprehensive multi-specialty patient nicotine replacement protocol, the hospital became smoke-free on inpatient, ambulatory, psychiatric, and long-term care grounds. The community has embraced the example set by these Magnet nurses, who now share their expertise to help other hospitals and organizations across the country go smoke-free.*

In another part of the country, nurses at Rochester General Hospital in Rochester, NY reported dissatisfaction with needle-less syringes. The staff council supervised a hospital-wide trial of four devices, convinced the Value Analysis Committee a change was necessary, and selected a system that was satisfactory to every specialty. Although the new system cost an additional $34,000 per year, needle-stick injuries dropped 26%, resulting in a net savings of $14,000. Nurses felt they were valued partners in achieving an important safety goal.

Transformational Front-line leaders

The significance of unit-level leadership, particularly that of nurse managers, is profound and directly impacts retention, staff decision-making, engagement, and innovation (Boyle et al., 1999; Laschinger, Finegan, & Wilk, 2009; Murphy, 2005). Unit leaders create a connected and committed workforce and cultivate innovation. At Virginia Commonwealth University Health System, a transformational nurse manager introduced a vision that had a significant impact on neonatal care in Central Virginia.

When the opportunity arose to transform the neonatal intensive care unit from one large room where premature and critically ill infants were cared for into a healing, nurturing, and technically sophisticated environment with all private rooms, nurse manager Sharon Cone, PhD(c), RN seized the opportunity. Cone involved the entire healthcare team and all ancillary support people in the design and construction of a new unit and building. Cone was able to move the staff from skepticism to a team that embraced a new vision and made it their own. After three years of planning, collaboration, and significant effort, a state-of-the-art facility opened and was the recipient of the General Electric Imagination at Work award for innovation. Success was measured by zero turnover, higher parent satisfaction, and very low hospital-acquired infections.

Advocacy and Influence of Nursing Executives

In Magnet organizations, the chief nursing officer influences organization-wide change. At NYU Hospitals Center, more than 90% of nurses are baccalaureate-educated. The medical center holds the distinction of employing one of the highest numbers of BSN-prepared nurses in the country. This is no coincidence. CNO Susan Bowar-Ferres, PhD, RN, in concert with her directors, incorporated educational preparation into the nursing strategic plan. Over the course of three years, with her team, Bowar-Ferres implemented a policy requiring a baccalaureate degree for all new nurses hired at the medical center. She also raised the education standard for nurse managers to the master's level, and made a doctorate the desired credential for clinical directors. To support these standards, Bowar-Ferres and her nurse leaders advocated for generous employee tuition reimbursement programs, which encouraged nurses to pursue advanced degrees.

SUMMARY

Transformational Leadership is purposeful and has the capacity to move an organization to greatness. Burns (1978) described transforming leadership as "dynamic in the sense that the leaders throw themselves into a relationship with followers who will feel 'elevated' by it and often become more active themselves" (p. 20). By understanding these transformational characteristics and how they impact staff and environment, leaders can create a culture of excellence and achieve Magnet designation. A transformational culture is formed through consistent trust, open communication, and strong relationships. Because transformational leaders are risk takers and change agents, some failure will undoubtedly occur. However, in a transformational culture, failure is viewed as a positive learning opportunity. As a result, innovation is always possible. Creating this transformational culture at every level is the key to success.

The future is uncertain, and nurse leaders will need to design and lead radically different models of health care. A shift from treating sickness to managing health and prevention will undoubtedly challenge our thinking about how patient care is delivered and how we focus our limited resources. Transformational nurse leaders will demonstrate their flexibility and adaptability within the framework of the Magnet Model. These pioneering leaders will work with great clinical staffs to create open and accessible structures and new patient care models that result in top clinical outcomes, ultimately improving the health of the nation. The Magnet organizations' nursing leadership is poised to manage the changes required, and it will be exciting to watch what the next generation brings to the future.

REFERENCES

All URLs retrieved September 12, 2010.

Aarons, G. A. (2006). Transformational and transactional leadership: Association with attitudes toward evidence-based practice. *Psychiatric Services, 57*(8), 1162–1169.

Armstrong, K., Laschinger, H., & Wong, C. (2009). Workplace empowerment and Magnet hospital characteristics as predictors of patient safety climate. *Journal of Nursing Administration, 24*(1), 55–62.

Atwater, L. E., & Yammarino, F. J. (1993). Personal attributes as predictors of superiors' and subordinates' perceptions of military academy leadership. *Human Relations, 46*, 645–668.

Avolio, B. J., Waldman, D. A., & Yammarino, F. J. (1991). Leading in the 1990s: The four L's of transformational leadership. *Journal of European Industrial Training, 15*(4), 9–16.

Bass, B. M. (1990). From transactional to transformational leadership: Learning to share the vision. *Organizational dynamics, 18*(3), 19–32.

Bass, B. M., Avolio, B. J., Jung, D. I., & Berson, Y. (2003). Predicting unit performance by assessing transformational and transactional Leadership. *Journal of Applied Psychology, 88*(2), 207–218.

Boyle, D. K., Bott, M. J., Woods, C. Q., Hansen, H. E., & Taunton, R. L. (1999). Managers' leadership and critical care nurses' intent to stay. *American Journal of Critical Care, 8*(6), 361–371.

Brady-Schwartz, D. C. (2005). Further evidence on the Magnet recognition program. *Journal of Nursing Administration, 35*(9), 397–403.

Burns, J. (1978). *Leadership.* New York, NY: Harper and Row.

Chan, K. Y., & Drasgow, F. (2001). Toward a theory of individual differences and leadership: Understanding the motivation to lead. *Journal of Applied Psychology, 86*(3), 481–498.

Chiok, F. L. (2001). Leadership behaviors: Effect on job satisfaction, productivity, and organizational commitment. *Journal of Nursing Management, 9*(4), 191–204.

Clarke, S. P. (2007). Hospital work environments, nurse characteristics, and sharps injuries. *American Journal of Infection Control, 35*(5), 302–309.

Dunham-Taylor, J. (2000). Nurse executive transformational leadership found in participative organizations. *Journal of Nursing Administration, 30*(5), 241–250.

Dunham-Taylor, J., & Klafehn, K. (1990). Transformational leadership and the nurse executive. *Journal of Nursing Administration, 20*(4), 28–34.

Failla, K. R., & Stichler, J. F. (2008). Manager and staff perceptions of the manager's leadership style. *Journal of Nursing Administration, 38*(11), 48–87.

Howell, J. M., & Avolio, B. J. (1993). Transformational leadership, transactional leadership, locus of control, and support for innovation: Key predictors of business unit performance. *Journal of Applied Psychology, 78*, 891–902.

Institute of Medicine (IOM). (2004). *Keeping patients safe: Transforming the work environment of nurses.* Washington, DC: Author

Kotter, J. P. (1996). *Leading change.* Boston, MA: Harvard Business School Press.

Kouzes, J. W., & Posner, B. Z. (1988). *The leadership challenge.* San Francisco, CA: Jossey-Bass Publishers.

Kramer, M., & Schmalenberg, C. (1988a). Magnet hospitals: Part I: Institutions of excellence. *Journal of Nursing Administration, 18*(1), 13–24.

Kramer, M., & Schmalenberg, C. (1988b). Magnet Hospitals: Part II: Institutions of excellence. *Journal of Nursing Administration, 18*(2), 11–19.

Laschinger, H. K., & Finegan, J. (2005). Using empowerment to build trust and respect in the workplace: A strategy for addressing the nursing shortage. *Nursing Economic$, 23*(1), 6–13.

Laschinger, H. K., Finegan, J., & Wilk, P. (2009). The impact of unit leadership and empowerment on nurses' organizational commitment. *Journal of Nursing Administration, 39*(5), 228–235.

Manojlovich, M., & Laschinger, H. (2007). The nursing worklife model: Extending and refining a new theory. *The Journal of Nursing Management, 15*(3), 256–263.

Muoro, G. (2009). American University of Beirut Medical Center. Retrieved from http://nursingservice. aub.edu.lb/users/index.asp

Murphy, L. (2005). Transformational leadership: A cascading chain reaction. *Journal of Nursing Management, 13*(2), 128–136.

Scott, J. G., Sochalski, J., & Aiken, L. (1999). Review of Magnet hospital research: Findings and implications for professional nursing practice. *Journal of Nursing Administration, 29*(1), 9–19.

Stordeur, S., Vandenberghe, C., & D'hoore, W. (2000). Leadership styles across hierarchical levels in nursing departments. *Nursing Research, 49*(1), 37–43.

Upenieks, V. V. (2003). What constitutes effective leadership? Perceptions of magnet and non-Magnet leaders. *Journal of Nursing Administration, 33*(9), 456–467.

Additional Resources

Aiken, L. H. (1995). Transformation of the nursing workforce. *Nursing Outlook, 43*, 201–209.

Altieri, L. (1995). *Transformational and transactional leadership in hospital nurse executives in the commonwealth of Pennsylvania: A descriptive study.* PhD dissertation. Fairfax, VA: George Mason University.

Anthony, M. K., Sauer, M. R., Standing, T. S., Sweeney, D. K., Glick, J., Modic, M. B., et al. (2005). Leadership and nurse retention: The pivotal role of nurse managers. *Journal of Nursing Administration, 35*(3), 146–155.

Aprigliano, T. (2000). The experience of courage development in transformational leaders. *Dissertation Abstracts International, 60*(10), 5245B.

Bass, B. M. (1985). *Leadership and performance beyond expectations.* New York, NY: Free Press

Buchan, J. M. (1999). Still attractive after all these years? Magnet hospitals in a changing health care environment. *Journal of Advanced Nursing, 30*(1), 100–108.

Calpin-Davies, P. (2000). Nurse manager, change thyself. *Nursing Management, 6*(9), 16–20.

Cameron, G. (1998). Transformational leadership: A strategy for organizational change. *Journal of Nursing Administration, 28*(10), 3.

Drenkard, K. N. (2005a). *The impact of transformational leadership characteristics of nurse managers on the anticipated turnover of RN staff nurses.* PhD dissertation. Fairfax, VA: George Mason Univ.

Drenkard, K. N. (2005b). Sustaining Magnet: Keeping the forces alive. *Nursing Administration Quarterly, 29*(3), 214–222.

Edmondson, A. C. (2003). Speaking up in the operating room: How team leaders promote learning in interdisciplinary action teams. *Journal of Management Studies, 40*(6), 1419–1452.

Edmondson, A. C. (2004). Psychological safety, trust, and learning: A group-level lens. In R. Kramer and K. Cook (Eds.), *Trust and distrust in organizations: Dilemmas and approaches,* pp. 239–272. New York: Russell Sage.

Edmondson, A. C., & Roloff, K. S. (2009). Overcoming barriers to collaboration: Psychological safety and learning in diverse teams. In E. Salas, G. F. Goodwin, and C. S. Burke (Eds.), *Team effectiveness in complex organizations: Cross-disciplinary perspectives and approaches,* pp. 183–208. New York, NY: Psychology Press.

Faulkner, J., & Laschinger, H. (2007). The effects of structural and psychological empowerment on perceived respect in acute care nurses. *Journal of Nursing Management, 16*, 214–221.

Furst, S. A., & Cable, D. M. (2008). Employee resistance to organizational change: Managerial influence tactics and leader-member exchange. *Journal of Applied Psychology, 93*(2), 453–462.

Girvin, J. (1996). Leadership and nursing: Part two: Styles of leadership. *Nursing Management, 3*(2), 20–21.

Judge, T. A., & Bono, J. E. (2000). Five factor model of personality and transformational leadership. *Journal of Applied Psychology, 85*(5), 751–765.

Kane-Urrabazo, C. K. (2006). Management's role in shaping organizational culture. *Journal of Nursing Management, 14,* 188–194.

Kanter, R. M. (1982). The middle manager as innovator. *Harvard Business Review, 60*(4), 95–105.

Kanter, R. M. (1993). *Men and women of the corporation* (2nd ed.). New York, NY: Basic Books.

Lake, E. (2002). Development of the practice environment scale of the nursing work index. *Research in Nursing & Health, 25,* 176–188.

Laschinger, H. K. S., Wong, C., McMahon, L., & Kaufman, C. (1999). Leader behavior impact on staff nurse empowerment, job tension, and work effectiveness. *Journal of Nursing Administration, 29*(5), 28–39.

Leach, L. S. (2005). Nurse executive transformational leadership and organizational commitment. *Journal of Nursing Administration, 35*(5), 228–237.

McClure, M. L., & Hinshaw, A. S. (2002). *Magnet hospitals revisited: Attraction and retention of professional nurses.* Washington, DC: American Nurses Publishing.

McDaniel, C., & Wolf, G. A. (1992). Transformational leadership in nursing service: A test of theory. *Journal of Nursing Administration, 22*(2), 60–65.

Meighan, M. M. (1990). The most important characteristics of nursing leaders. *Nursing Administration Quarterly, 15*(1), 63–69.

Moore, S. C., & Hutchinson, S. A. (2007). Developing leaders at every level. *Journal of Nursing Administration, 37*(12), 564–568.

Morrison, R., Jones, S., & Fuller, B. (1997). The relation between leadership style and empowerment on job satisfaction of nurses. *Journal of Nursing Administration, 27*(5), 27–34.

Murphy, L. (2005). Transformational leadership: A cascading chain reaction. *Journal of Nursing Management, 13*(2), 128–136.

Northouse, P. G. (2007). *Leadership: Theory and practice* (4th ed.). Thousand Oaks, CA: Sage Publications.

Perra, B. M. (2000). Leadership: The key to quality outcomes. *Nursing Administration Quarterly, 24*(2), 56–61.

Porter, A. H. (2009). AUB Medical Center designated first. Retrieved from http://www.aub.edu.lb/news/archive/preview.php?id=96941

Schein, E. H. (1985). *Organizational culture and leadership.* San Francisco, CA: Jossey-Bass.

Schein, E. H., & Bennis, W. (1965). *Personal and organizational change through group methods.* New York, NY: Wiley.

Scoble, K. B., & Russell, G. (2003). Vision 2020, Part I: Profile of the future nurse leader. *Journal of Nursing Administration, 33*(6), 324–330.

Sieloff, C. L. (2003). Leadership behaviors that foster nursing group power. *Journal of Nursing Management, 12*(4), 246–251.

Turner, N., Barling, J., Epitropaki, O., Butcher, V., & Milner, C. (2002). Transformational leadership and moral reasoning. *Journal of Applied Psychology, 87*(2), 304–311.

Ward, K. (2002). A vision for tomorrow: Transformational nursing leaders. *Nursing Outlook, 50*(30), 121–126.

Way, C., Lefort, S., Gregory, D., Barrett, B., Davis, J., Parfrey, P., et al. (2007). The impact of organizational culture on clinical managers' organizational commitment and turnover intentions. *Journal of Nursing Administration, 37*(5), 235–242.

Wolf, G., Boland, S., & Aukerman, M. (1994). A transformational model for the practice of nursing: Part 1, the model. *Journal of Nursing Administration, 24*(4), 51–57.

Wolf, G., Bradle, J., & Nelson, G. (2005). Bridging the strategic leadership gap: A model program for transformational change. *Journal of Nursing Administration, 35*(2), 54–60.

5

Structural Empowerment

Lois L. Kercher, PhD, RN
Janet Y. Harris, MSN, RN, NEA-BC

Every French soldier carries a marshal's baton in his knapsack.
Napoleon

The leader builds dispersed and diverse leadership—distributing leadership to the outermost edges of the circle to unleash the power of shared responsibility.
Frances Hesselbein

INTRODUCTION

Structural Empowerment is the Magnet® model component that addresses how the workplace environment supports exemplary professional practice, new knowledge, and improved outcomes. This chapter begins with a detailed look at the terms involved and then examines the component's five subcategories:

- Professional Engagement
- Commitment to Professional Development
- Teaching and Role Development
- Commitment to Community Involvement
- Recognition of Nursing

The relationship of these workplace characteristics to improved organizational performance is examined through the literature, research, and examples of exemplary practice in Magnet-designated settings. This is the "evidence" behind Structural Empowerment's "Sources of Evidence" as delineated in the Magnet Model. These characteristics were identified in the original study of Magnet hospitals (McClure et al., 1983). Ongoing studies from the healthcare industry, and the business world in general, continue to demonstrate their importance to a healthy workplace, high performance, and positive outcomes.

STRUCTURE AND ITS RELATIONSHIP TO QUALITY

Evaluation of quality in health care has long been approached using a conceptual framework with three elements: structure, process, and outcomes. The importance of this triad was first described in 1980 by Avedis Donabedian, considered the primary architect of the study of quality in healthcare services.

Structure includes the conditions under which care is provided. It encompasses organizational, human, environmental, and physical resources. Policies, procedures, systems, and programs are part of structure. *Process* includes activities, interventions, and the sequence of events that constitute care giving. *Outcomes*, the ultimate indicator of quality, are the consequences to the patient's health that are dependent on structure and process. Donabedian's formula, in which structure and process are pivotal in producing a desired outcome, has driven the evaluation of healthcare quality for more than 30 years. The Magnet Model incorporates this conceptual framework.

THE MEANING OF EMPOWERMENT

Empowerment is defined as "the giving or delegation of power or authority; the giving of an ability, enablement or permission" (Collins, 2003). Within the Magnet environment, it refers to the way in which transformational leaders develop, direct, enable, and reward direct care nurses to perform at their highest level of practice and achieve autonomy in patient care. These leaders generally create flat management structures that facilitate vertical communication and maximize involvement of point-of-care staff. Empowering nurses in the workplace requires that they have the resources and opportunity to drive exemplary practice and outcomes. Empowered nurses influence decisions and, in a culture of accountability, are responsible for the resulting outcomes. As a Magnet Model component, *Structural Empowerment* refers to an organization designed to foster engagement of nurses in their professional practice both internally and externally. Priorities include perpetual learning and promotion of nurses as teachers. Community involvement is encouraged and enabled. Nursing's positive image in a Magnet setting is palpable.

PROFESSIONAL ENGAGEMENT

A Magnet hospital must demonstrate that nurses from all settings and roles are involved in organizational decisions. Why is this internal engagement important? The rationale stems from the science of management. Studies of all types of organizations, including health care, show that involving employees in operational decisions improves production, performance, and outcomes. (Armstrong et al., 2009; Gallup, 2006; Golanowski et al., 2007; Schneider et al., 2009).

The value of partnering with employees in organizational decisions emerged during the latter half of the twentieth century. Prior to that, management theories were based on models of centralized authority, layers of hierarchy, and rigid channels of communication. When behavioral scientists began to study human behavior in organizations, they discovered the importance of leadership style, teamwork, and engagement of personnel (Koontz et al., 1984).

One of the most notable contributors to the field of organizational performance is Rosabeth Moss Kanter, who conducted a five-year, in-depth analysis of the anatomy and culture of a major corporation (1977). Kanter found that organizational success is associated with an empowered workforce where employees are engaged. According to Kanter, this empowerment occurs when four conditions are present:
- Employees have access to information.
- They have adequate resources to do their job.
- They are supported by feedback from management and peers.
- They have the opportunity to learn and grow.

Kanter's theory has been tested in a number of nursing studies and the results confirm a relationship between an empowered nursing staff and improvements in the workplace (Cho et al., 2006; Kramer et al., 2008; Laschinger & Finegan, 2005; Mangold et al., 2006; Patrick & Laschinger, 2006). There is clear evidence supporting the value of engaging staff. This work has been further supported by the work of the Gallup Organization. Research has demonstrated that a more engaged nursing staff leads to better outcomes and involvement in decision-making (Gallup Organization, 2006). In addition, Gallup has shared data that Magnet hospital nurses are more engaged than nurses in hospitals that are not Magnet (Drenkard, 2010).

Creating a workplace setting where nurses are empowered requires transformational leaders who understand their management responsibilities. Nursing leaders need to develop an infrastructure where direct care nurses are involved in decisions. There are challenges to achieving a culture of engagement. Changes in health care occur at a rapid pace. This means nurses need to devote time participating in decisions about practice changes. The need to control healthcare costs often reduces the opportunity for direct care nurses to be paid for hours in meetings collaborating with peers. Another challenge to peer collaboration comes as a result of expansion of hospitals into systems. This increases the number of nurses who need to be involved in standardizing policy and procedure, and these nurses may work in settings far from each other. Fortunately, new technologies will enable nurses to participate in operational and practice decisions even when they cannot meet face to face.

The future of electronic discussion capability, social networking, and online interactivity will transform the ability of Magnet organizations to connect with all staff within the organization. The future of communication and collaboration across workplace boundaries lies in electronic and online knowledge networking. New types of software enable team members to connect virtually through a network (Sampson, 2009). People can remotely share knowledge, respond to problems, participate in decisions, and generate innovation without physically gathering together in the same room. Nursing leaders need to develop expertise in this technology and support direct care nurses in the use of knowledge networking (MacPhee et al., 2009). The future is limitless with regard to connectivity, and new ways of communicating and participating will grow exponentially over the next decade. Creative leaders look to leverage the possible connections and incorporate them into the structures of the organization.

External engagement is equally important, and nurses at Magnet facilities are expected to be involved in professional organizations outside the hospital walls. Benefits of professional organizations include:
- Development of professional standards
- Forum for networking and sharing knowledge
- Opportunity for individual professional development
- Public education
- Consumer protection
- Advocacy to advance the profession's mission and vision

The American Nurses Association (ANA) began in 1896. The first International Council of Nurses was formed in 1905 with the United States, Great Britain, and Germany as members (ANA web site). Today, nurses are connected through myriad professional organizations, some broad in their mission and vision, others targeted to a narrow subspecialty of nursing practice. Nurses are involved at the local, regional, state, national, and international levels. Engagement in professional nursing organizations brings value to individual nursing practice, nursing performance within an organization, the profession at large, and society. It dovetails with Magnet's vision to "lead the reformation of health care; the discipline of nursing; and care of the patient, family, and community." Active membership in professional associations is one way nurses turn this vision into reality. Nurses in Magnet hospitals realize the advantages of working together across boundaries and through their professional organizations. In Virginia, a Consortium of Magnet Hospitals was convened with leadership from the Virginia Nurses Association. These organizations meet regularly to share best practices and work together across the state to improve patient care.

COMMITMENT TO PROFESSIONAL DEVELOPMENT

In 1964, ANA established that a baccalaureate degree in nursing (BSN) was the minimum preparation necessary for beginning professional nursing practice (ANA web site). More than four decades later, nursing has yet to achieve this goal. Historically, one of the drivers for advancing baccalaureate education was to ensure credible professional identity for nursing compared to other clinical disciplines. Now, an even greater imperative drives the requirement that nurses have a BSN to practice. Research findings show a positive relationship between the practice of baccalaureate-prepared nurses and desired patient outcomes (Aiken et al., 2003).

In a major study of over 230,000 surgical patients cared for in 168 hospitals, each 10% increase in the proportion of nurses with a BSN or higher degree was associated with a 5% lower risk of mortality and failure to rescue (Aiken et al., 2003). Similar results were found in a study of 18,000 patients in 49 hospitals in Canada (Estabrooks et al., 2005). Another study in Canada found a 10% increase in proportion of baccalaureate-prepared nurses was associated with nine fewer deaths for every 1,000 discharged patients (Tourangeau et al., 2007). In a longitudinal study of 21 U.S. hospitals over 84 quarters, nurse researchers found hospitals with a higher proportion of BSN-educated nurses had lower rates of congestive heart failure mortality, hospital-acquired pressure ulcers, and failure to rescue, as well as shorter inpatient length of stay (Blegen & Goode, 2010). Research has shown that adverse patient outcomes are often associated with lack of critical thinking. Baccalaureate education prepares nurses to use critical thinking skills in synthesizing complex clinical information. This is essential for reliable delivery of quality patient care.

A major study released by the Carnegie Institute calls for a radical transformation in the education of the nursing profession and a requirement for BSN as entry into practice (Benner et al., 2010). The Tri-Council for Nursing, which includes the American Association of Colleges of Nursing, the American Nurses Association, the American Organization of Nurse Executives, and the National League for Nursing, is united in the view that a more highly educated nursing workforce is critical to meeting the nation's nursing needs and delivering safe, effective patient care (ANA, 2010).

The Magnet Recognition Program® began specifying education credentials in 2005, but only for the chief nursing officer (CNO), who was required to have a master's degree. Another requirement for the CNO was added in January 2008, specifying the CNO needed either a baccalaureate or master's degree in nursing. With greater evidence now placed on outcomes, and mounting evidence linking patient outcomes and educational preparation, nurses in Magnet organizations must increasingly be educated at the baccalaureate level and higher. The first step is to require that front-line clinical nurse leaders have a minimum of a baccalaureate degree in the profession. The future for the Magnet Recognition Program will be to base the Sources of Evidence on research and evidence-based findings, and this growing research will continue to inform the requirements for nursing excellence.

The Magnet manual published in 2008 specifies, "Effective January 1, 2011, 75% of nurse managers of individual units/wards/clinics must have at least a baccalaureate degree in nursing upon submission of the application. By January 1, 2013, 100% of nurse managers of individual units/wards/clinics must have at least a baccalaureate degree in nursing upon submission of the application" (ANCC, 2008). As research continues to demonstrate a relationship between patient outcomes and educational preparation, it should be anticipated that more nurses in Magnet organizations will be educated at the baccalaureate level and higher to assure quality patient outcomes.

Healthcare organizations seeking Magnet designation must demonstrate support for professional nursing certification. This includes setting goals for the number of nurses certified, and helping nurses achieve these goals. Why is certification of value? According to the National Organization for Competency Assurance, "certification represents a declaration of a particular individual's professional competence" (Institute for Credentialing Excellence, 2010).

Among physicians, specialty certification is an expected credential. At a minimum, they must have it to receive hospital privileges and reimbursement from insurance companies. There are several studies that show a positive correlation between physicians' certification status and desired patient care processes and outcomes (Chen et al., 2006; Miller et al., 2004). Studies also show a relationship between internists who score high on their certification examination and improved management of patient care (Norcini et al., 2002).

It seems logical to support professional nursing certification among registered nurses for similar reasons. But what is known about the relationship between certified nurses and patient outcomes? The answer is emerging as studies begin to address this question. Although the findings are not yet conclusive, there is preliminary evidence of a positive correlation between nurses who are certified and their level of practice.

In comparisons of the performance of certified and non-certified nurses, those who were certified scored higher in patient care planning and evaluation (Redd & Alexander, 1997). In a study of 19,452 nurses, those who had achieved certification reported that it improved their confidence in identifying complications and initiating effective intervention (Cary, 2001). This same study found that 40% of nurses certified five years or less reported experiencing fewer errors in patient care which they attributed to knowledge gained from certification (Cary, 2001). The National Quality Forum (NQF, 2008) has identified failure to rescue hospitalized patients from a rapid decline in their clinical condition as a nurse-sensitive measure of quality of care. Studies have found that certified nurses are more likely to conduct frequent assessments for cues that their patients need urgent intervention to avoid demise (Clarke & Aiken, 2003).

Nurses with hospice certification performed significantly better in delivering respiratory care than their non-certified counterparts as measured by the correct use of nebulizer therapy (Scarpaci et al., 2007). Correct classification of pressure ulcers was more likely if the nurse was certified in the specialty (Hart et al., 2006). Research on patient safety in critical care units demonstrated that the greater the percentage of certified nurses, the lower the rate of patient falls (Kendall-Gallagher & Blegen, 2009). A chart audit of oncology patients found nurses who were specialty-certified followed evidence-based practice for management of chemotherapy-induced nausea and vomiting more often than nurses without the certification (Coleman et al., 2009).

As research continues to demonstrate a relationship between patient outcomes and certification, it should be anticipated that more nurses in Magnet organizations will seek certification to ensure quality patient outcomes. In addition, the public is increasingly requiring evidence of competency in healthcare professionals, and certification is a measure of competence and knowledge attainment.

Early in the history of nursing, Florence Nightingale recognized the need for nurses to continually update and refresh their knowledge and skills. She would be amazed at the array of new knowledge and information available to the nurse today, and the dazzling array and access of information will only continue to grow. Nightingale supported the notion that all healthcare professionals, including nurses, need ongoing education to keep abreast of new knowledge in their specialty. Continuing education is also important for acquisition of skills needed for a new role or a change in responsibilities. Magnet organizations are expected to develop and provide continuing education programs for nurses. More importantly, they need to measure the effectiveness of these programs.

How is the effectiveness of an educational experience evaluated? Traditionally, evaluation forms have included these basic questions assessing the participant's reaction to the program: Was the content clear, and were the objectives of the program met? Did the speaker communicate well, and were audiovisual aids helpful? Was the room comfortable and was the food acceptable? These conditions may be important for learning to occur, but evaluation of any program should also ask the next level of query, that is, did learning occur? Sometimes this is measured through pre-test and post-test. A more sophisticated measure of the effectiveness of an educational program, however, is whether knowledge was transferred, and subsequently resulted in changing the practice or performance of the participant. This is harder to measure, but an attempt should be made to evaluate change in behavior due to new knowledge.

Ultimately, the goal of an educational program is to enable the participant to improve performance and deliver results. The desired impact of education should be improved outcomes related to the participants' change in behavior. A continuing education program for nurses ideally will lead to improved healthcare outcomes for patients. Four levels of assessing training effectiveness—reactions, learning, transfer, and results—are known as Kirkpatrick's Four Levels of Evaluation (Winfrey, 1999). Magnet organizations should strive to evaluate the effectiveness of their nursing educational programs using all four levels of assessment.

Newer methods of instruction, including computer-based training and simulation experience, have great potential for improving the ability to measure the effectiveness of education. These methods will enhance our ability to evaluate change in behavior concurrent with or immediately following instruction.

Magnet organizations are expected to take an active role in providing career development opportunities for people who seek to become a professional nurse. Predictions of a nursing shortage have been well documented (Buerhaus et al., 2006). The responsibility to ensure an adequate supply of nurses, and other healthcare professionals, belongs to society at large. Magnet organizations, as champions of the Magnet vision, have a unique responsibility to ensure there are adequate numbers of nurses to meet future community needs. As Magnet organizations seek to attract and retain nurses to their setting, so should they also actively attract prospective nurses into the profession.

The American Hospital Association (AHA) offers a toolkit describing how hospital leaders can build a thriving workforce (AHA, 2002). The recommendations include five key areas of activity:
- Foster meaningful work by designing all aspects of work around patients and the needs of staff.
- Improve the workplace partnership to value and engage all hospital staff.
- Broaden the base by creating a more diverse workforce.
- Collaborate with the broader community to attract new entrants into health care.
- Build societal support to ensure adequate resources for the healthcare system.

One of the tactical recommendations in the AHA toolkit, under the category of fostering meaningful work, is to "embrace the characteristics of the Magnet hospital program and incorporate them in work innovation" (AHA, 2002, p. 18). The AHA toolkit also describes numerous programs designed to support new entrants into healthcare careers. Many of the examples illustrate how hospitals across the country provide career development opportunities for non-nurse employees and members of the community interested in becoming nurses (AHA, 2002, p. 27).

TEACHING AND ROLE DEVELOPMENT

The original research on Magnet found that direct care nurses were very active as teachers (McClure et al., 1983, p. 94). Education of patients and family members was cited as providing job satisfaction for the nurses. Nurses viewed education of peers and other clinical staff as a fulfillment of their professional responsibility. Teaching was also seen by nurses as a means to advance their own competencies.

The role of nurses in teaching patients is prescribed in the scope of practice of the profession. ANA's standards of practice for nursing include a criterion that nurses employ strategies to promote health and a safe environment (ANA, 2010, p. 36). Teaching patients is integral to the process of nursing. Patient-centeredness is one of the six aims of quality care proposed by the Institute of Medicine (IOM, 2004). Among the characteristics of patient-centered care is healthcare information in language that people understand. They need information about (1) how to stay well, or what is wrong with them, (2) what is likely to happen and how they will be affected, and (3) what can be done to change or manage their condition. As patients become more active partners in their own health care, the teaching role of the nurse gains significance.

It is also incumbent upon nurses, as professionals, to engage in teaching peers. The ANA standards of professional performance address nurses' responsibility to share knowledge and skills by teaching peers and colleagues (ANA, 2010, p. 49). Magnet-designated hospitals create opportunities for direct care nurses to participate in teaching others within their organization, and also in the nursing community at large. Nurses in a hospital recognized by the Magnet program are expected to serve as mentors to colleagues in other organizations who pursue the Magnet journey.

Partnership models between hospitals and schools of nursing vary considerably across the United States. Most hospitals serve as clinical sites for nursing students, and some have agreements for adjunct faculty, scholarship support, research collaboration, and shared resources such as simulation technology or libraries. Magnet-designated Providence Portland Medical Center and the University of Portland in Oregon, have developed an exemplary model for partnership between academe and service. Through the initiation of dedicated education units, the organization provides staff nurses as clinical faculty during clinical rotations, and the academic faculty coach educates the staff nurses to increase their clinical teaching skills. The dedicated education units have been so successful that the University of Portland School of Nursing, in conjunction with the organization, has been awarded a Robert Wood Johnson grant to evaluate this innovative approach to expand teaching capacity (Warner & Burton, 2009). The future will most likely include deeper relationships between academic institutions and healthcare organizations, as learning becomes lifelong and career progressions move to integrate the role of nurse as teacher and practitioner of clinical nursing care. Future creative partnerships may see blending of service and academic roles, better integration of nursing research activities into clinical care, and sharing of scarce physical resources such as simulation labs and human resources such as specialized nurse clinicians.

Nurses who complete their education and successfully pass their licensing examination embark upon a critical period in their professional life known as entry into practice. Much has been written about this period of role transition from student to professional nurse. Research has shown that the initial year of practice after graduation is characterized by disillusionment and high attrition. Magnet organizations are expected to effectively manage entry into practice and must describe how they facilitate the transition of the new graduate into the work environment.

New nursing graduates enter the workplace with a wide variety of skill level and preparation. Their readiness for practice is based on many factors, including the type of instruction and clinical experience they received as students. Regardless of how well their education prepared them for practice, nurses progress through distinct phases of sequential skill acquisition once they begin to deliver patient care. Dreyfus, who studied chess players and airline pilots, initially described the phenomenon of gradual acquisition of skill through practice (Dreyfus & Dreyfus, 1980). The Dreyfus Model postulates five levels of ability, each characterized as follows:

1. **Novice:** rigid adherence to rules; no discretional judgment
2. **Advanced Beginner:** situational perception still limited
3. **Competent:** partially sees action as part of longer-term goals; conscious deliberate planning
4. **Proficient:** holistic view of the situation; uses maxims for guidance
5. **Expert:** intuitive grasp of situation, based on tacit knowledge

Benner applied the Dreyfus Model to nursing (Benner, 1984). According to Benner, new graduate nurses are not the only novices in the practice setting. Nurses in a clinical area where they have no experience with the specialty or patient population may be novices in that setting.

COMMITMENT TO COMMUNITY INVOLVEMENT

Magnet healthcare organizations are role-models in fostering improved community health. The recipient of the Magnet Prize Award in 2009, Poudre Valley Hospital of Fort Collins, CO, goes beyond its front doors to strengthen the health of the most vulnerable individuals in its community. The hospital's Community Case Management Program serves individuals who often have no other options—primarily the low-income, elderly, and chronically ill. "Each year, close to 400 clients receive one-on-one services at no charge from advanced practice nurses. Nurses enter clients' homes to improve their functioning and life circumstances. Clients receive at least three visits or calls each month. Through this constant care, a strong, therapeutic relationship is formed and health is stabilized and improved. The number of times a client is admitted to the hospital or visits the emergency department declines significantly. Clients report feeling more at ease and effective at managing their chronic conditions and their lives. Fully financially supported by the hospital, this program is independently run by advanced practice nurses and a master's-level licensed clinical social worker. It serves long- and short-term patients without time or disease limits, it has sustained costs savings to the institution which significantly surpass the cost of the program, and it has a proven track record after fifteen successful years. The concepts guiding the Poudre Valley Community Case Management Program have the potential to transform nursing practice and health care nationally. It reflects the focus of today's healthcare reform where reducing costs, increasing access to health care, and managing chronic diseases are priorities" (Poudre Valley Hospital, ANCC, 2009).

RECOGNITION OF NURSING

The significance of nursing to the mission and the vision of the organization is overtly recognized in a Magnet setting. Recognition of the contribution of nurses is built into the structure and process of operations. It ranges from praise for individual performance to facility-wide recognition of the value of nursing. In a study of more than 400 companies, praising people for doing good work was identified as one of 12 key behaviors used by managers to attract and retain the most talented workforce (Buckingham & Coffman, 1999). Research has shown that improved organizational performance is associated with a 5:1 ratio in giving positive and negative feedback. For each comment of constructive criticism, there should be five comments of praise.

In addition to acknowledging individual and team performance, it is important to recognize the clinical discipline of professional nursing for the value it brings to healthcare quality. As stated in a report of the Institute of Medicine:

> "When we are hospitalized, … —at some of our most vulnerable moments—nurses are the healthcare providers we are most likely to encounter, spend the greatest amount of time with, and be dependent upon for recovery. Nursing actions such as ongoing monitoring of patient health status have been shown to be directly related to better patient outcomes." (IOM, 2004, Foreword, ix)

Healthcare facilities need to value all of the members of the organization for the unique role each person plays in the delivery of care. This is emphasized in the Force of Magnetism emphasizing interdisciplinary relationships. However, professional nurses are pivotal to teamwork and their contribution to patient care should be highlighted. Magnet organizations are those that recognize and make visible the contributions of nursing to patient care. Nursing's positive image in a Magnet setting is palpable.

It is expected that a Magnet-designated facility, or system, is known for excellence in patient care. The organization should be associated with high-quality outcomes and contribution to the local community and beyond. A Magnet organization has an exemplary reputation.

The Magnet manual (2008) states that "in the interest of advancing the nursing profession, Magnet organizations are expected to mentor others." This includes sharing their Magnet journey experience with other hospitals. Nurses from Magnet hospitals should be active in disseminating their best practice through poster presentations, speaking at professional meetings, and publishing. This activity is essential if Magnet organizations are to serve as the fount of knowledge and expertise for the delivery of nursing care globally and lead the reformation of health care; the discipline of nursing; and care of the patient, family, and community.

SUMMARY

Delivery of healthcare service is becoming ever more challenging as the healthcare system grows more complex and the demand for service escalates. Nursing plays a critical role in addressing these challenges as the single largest provider of the healthcare workforce. In the future, evidence-based work retention models that enable decisions to be made closest to the patient, that support professional development and value staff, must be implemented across the board. Building and maintaining a structure where nurse autonomy can flourish will yield positive patient outcomes. These structures will continue to evolve and be influenced by advances in technology, changes in financial methodologies, and the needs of nurses in a positive workplace.

REFERENCES

All URLs retrieved September 12, 2010.

Aiken, L., Clarke, S., Cheung, R., Sloane, D., & Silber, J. (2003). Educational levels of hospital nurses and surgical patient mortality. *Journal of the American Medical Association, 290*(12), 1617–1623.

American Hospital Association. (2002). *In our hands: How hospital leaders can build a thriving workforce. Report of the AHA Commission on Workforce for Hospitals and Health Systems.* Washington, DC: Author. Retrieved from http://www.aha.org/aha/resource-center/Statistics-and-Studies/ioh.html

American Nurses Association. (2000). ANA reaffirms commitment to BSN for entry into practice. Retrieved from http://www.nursingworld.org/FunctionalMenuCategories/MediaResources/PressReleases/2000/CommitmenttoBSN.aspx

American Nurses Association. (2007). Basic historical review of nursing and the ANA. Retrieved from http://www.nursingworld.org/FunctionalMenuCategories/AboutANA/WhoWeAre/History.aspx

American Nurses Association. (2010). *Nursing: Scope and standards of practice, 2nd edition.* Silver Spring, MD: Author.

American Nurses Association. (2010). Tri-Council for Nursing issues new consensus policy statement on the educational advancement of registered nurses. Retrieved from http://www.nursingworld.org/FunctionalMenuCategories/MediaResources/PressReleases/2010-PR/TriCouncil-for-Nursing-Issues-Policy-Statement.aspx

American Nurses Credentialing Center. (2008). *Application manual: Magnet Recognition Program.* Silver Spring, MD: Author.

American Nurses Credentialing Center. (2009). Magnet prize award application, internal document. Silver Spring, MD: Author.

Armstrong, K., Laschinger, H., & Wong, C. (2009). Workplace empowerment and Magnet hospital characteristics as predictors of patient safety climate. *Journal of Nursing Administration, 39*(7/8), S17-S24.

Benner, P. (1984). *From novice to expert: Excellence and power in clinical nursing practice.* Menlo Park, CA: Addison-Wesley.

Benner, P., Sutphen, M., Leonard, V., & Day, L. (2010). *Educating nurses: A call for radical transformation.* San Francisco, CA: Jossey-Bass.

Blegen, M., & Goode, C. (2010). Nurse staffing and quality of care—Effects on BSN education. Indianapolis, IN: Presentation at the American Organization of Nurse Executives 43rd Annual Meeting and Exposition.

Buckingham, M., & Coffman, C. (1999). *First break all the rules: What the world's greatest managers do differently.* New York, NY: Simon & Schuster.

Buerhaus, P., Donelan, K., Ulrich, B., Norman, L., & Dittus, R. (2006). State of the registered nurse workforce in the United States. *Nursing Economic$, 24*(1), 6–12.

Cary, A. H. (2001). Certified registered nurses: Results of the study of the certified workforce. *American Journal of Nursing, 101*(1), 44–52.

Chen, J., Rathore, S. S., Wang, Y., Radford, M. J., & Krumholz, H. M. (2006). Physician board certification and the care and outcomes of elderly patients with acute myocardial infarction. *Journal of General Internal Medicine, 21*(3), 238–244.

Cho, J., Laschinger, Laschinger, H. K., & Wong, C. (2006). Workplace empowerment, work engagement and organizational commitment of new graduate nurses. *Nursing Leadership, 19*(3), 43–60.

Clarke, S. P., & Aiken, L. (2003). Failure to rescue: Needless deaths are prime examples of the need for more nurses at the bedside. *American Journal of Nursing, 103*(1), 42–47.

Coleman, E. A., Coon, S. K., Lockhart, K., Kennedy, R. L., Montgomery, R., Copeland, N., . . . Stewart, C. (2009). Effect of certification in oncology nursing on nursing-sensitive outcomes. *Clinical Journal of Oncology Nursing, 13*(2), 165–171.

Collins English Dictionary: Complete and unabridged 10th edition. (2003). New York, NY: Harper Collins Publishers. Retrieved from http://dictionary.reference.com/browse/empowerment.

Donabedian, A. (1980). *Explorations in quality assessment and monitoring, vol. I: The definition of quality and approaches to its assessment.* Ann Arbor, MI: Health Administration Press.

Drenkard, K. (2010). Going for the gold: The value of attaining Magnet recognition. *American Nurse Today, 5*(3), 50–52.

Dreyfus, H. L., & Dreyfus, S. (1980). *A five-stage model of the mental activities involved in directed skill acquisition.* Berkeley, CA: Operations Research Center, University of California.

http://dictionary.reference.com/browse/empowerment

Estabrooks, C., Midodzi, W. K., Cummings, G., Ricker, K., & Giovannetti, P. (2005). The impact of hospital nursing characteristics on 30-day mortality. *Nursing Research, 54*(2), 74–84.

Gallup Organization. (2006). Gallup study: Engaged employees inspire company innovation. *Gallup Management Journal.* (October 12.) Retrieved from http://gmj.gallup.com/content/24880/gallup-study-engaged-employees-inspire-company.aspx

Golanowski, M., Beaudry, D., Kurz, L., Laffey, W. J., & Hook, M. L. (2007). Interdisciplinary shared decision-making: Taking shared governance to the next level. *Nursing Administration Quarterly, 31*(4), 341–353.

Hart, S., Bergquist, S., Gajewski, B., & Dunton, N. (2006). Reliability testing of the national database of nursing quality indicators pressure ulcer indicator. *Journal of Nursing Care Quality, 21*(3), 256–265.

Institute for Credentialing Excellence. (2010) What is Certification? Washington, DC: Author. Retrieved from http://www.credentialingexcellence.org/GeneralInformation/WhatisCertification/tabid/63/Default.aspx.

Institute of Medicine of the National Academies of Science. (2004). *Keeping patients safe: Transforming the work environment of nurses.* Washington, DC: The National Academies Press.

Kanter, R. M. (1977). *Men and women of the corporation.* New York, NY: Basic Books.

Kendall-Gallagher, D., & Blegen, M. A. (2009). Competence and certification of registered nurses and safety of patients in intensive care units. *American Journal of Critical Care, 18,* 106–113.

Koontz, H. D., O'Donnell, C., & Weihrich, H. (1984). *Management.* New York, NY: McGraw-Hill.

Kramer, M., Schmalenberg, C., Maguire, P., Brewer, B., Burke, R., Chmielewski, L.,. . . Waldo, M. (2008). Structures and practices enabling staff nurses to control their practice. *Western Journal of Nursing Research, 30*(5), 539–559.

Laschinger, H. K., & Finegan, J. (2005). Empowering nurses for work engagement and health in hospital settings. *Journal of Nursing Administration, 35*(10), 439–449.

MacPhee, M., Suryaprakash, N., & Jackson, C. (2009). Online knowledge networking. *Journal of Nursing Administration, 39*(10), 415–422.

Mangold, K. L., Pearson, K. K., Schmitz, J. R., Scherb, C. A., Specht, J. P., & Loes, J. L. (2006). Perceptions and characteristics of registered nurses' involvement in decision-making. *Nursing Administration Quarterly, 30*(3), 266–272.

McClure, M. L., Poulin, M., Sovie, M., & Wandelt, M. (1983). *Magnet hospitals: Attraction and retention of professional nurses.* Kansas City, MO: American Nurses Association.

Miller, G., Britt, H., Pan, Y., & Knox, S. (2004). Relationship between general practitioner certification and characteristics of care. *Medical Care, 42*(8), 770–778.

National Quality Forum. (2004). *National voluntary consensus standards for nursing-sensitive care: An initial performance measure set.* Washington, DC: Author.

National Quality Forum. (2008). Home page accessed at http://www.qualityforum.org.

Norcini, J. J., Lipner, R., & Kimball, H. (2002). Certifying examination performance and patient outcomes following myocardial infarction. *Medical Education, 36*(9), 853–859.

Patrick, A., & Laschinger, H. K. (2006). The effect of structural empowerment and perceived organizational support on middle-level nurse managers' role satisfaction. *Journal of Nursing Management, 14*(1), 13–22.

Poudre Valley Hospital 2009 Magnet Prize Award Application. (Unpublished internal document.) Silver Spring, MD: American Nurses Credentialing Center.

Redd, M. L., & Alexander, J. W. (1977). Does certification mean better performance? *Nursing Management, 28*(2), 45–49.

Sampson, M. (2009). *Seamless teamwork: Using Microsoft® SharePoint® Technologies to collaborate, innovate, and drive business in new ways.* Redmond, WA: Microsoft Press.

Scarpaci, L. T., Tsoukleris, M. G., & McPherson, M. L. (2007). Assessment of hospice nurses' technique in the use of inhalers and nebulizers. *Journal of Palliative Medicine, 10*(3), 665–676.

Schneider, B., Stacey, W. H., Barbera, K. M., & Martin, N. (2009). Driving customer satisfaction and financial success through employee engagement. *People & Strategy, 32*(2), 23–27.

Tourangeau, A. E., Doran, D. M., Hall, L., Obrien-Pallas, L., Pringle, D., Tu, J. V., & Cranley, L. A. (2007). Impact of hospital nursing care on 30-day mortality for acute medical patients. *Journal of Advanced Nursing, 57*(1), 32–44.

Warner, J., & Burton, D. (2009). The policy and politics of emerging academic-service partnerships. *Journal of Professional Nursing, 25*(6), 329–334.

Winfrey, E. C. (1999). Kirkpatrick's four levels of evaluation. In B. Hoffman (Ed.), *Encyclopedia of educational technology.* Retrieved from http://edweb.sdsu.edu/eet/articles/k4levels/start.htm

6

Exemplary Professional Practice

Patricia Reid-Ponte, DNSc, RN, NEA-BC, FAAN
Angela Creta, MS, RN, CNL-BC
Christina Joy, DNSc, RN

What if I am exactly what is needed at this time for this patient?
Dr. Rachel Naomi Remen

Knowing is not enough, we must apply; willing is not enough, we must do.
Goethe

A professional nursing practice that is considered "exemplary" must be designed, implemented, and advanced over time. It needs an explicit and observable set of values and philosophies, as well as practical methods for conducting work, setting priorities, and making decisions. It requires transformational leadership, strategic direction, the proper infrastructure and resources, and a solid set of operational plans and processes. It also must include a system for looking inward and outward that is self-reflective, continuous, and able to detect best practices that may be emerging elsewhere. New knowledge and changing external demands, regulations, and policy require that leaders and staff have a dependable method for learning, monitoring, and continuously improving based on evolving evidence. Such a practice is steeped in the deepest behaviors of respect, collaboration, fairness, and justice. It highly values diversity of opinion, thought, and ethnicity.

This chapter provides an in-depth description of these practice elements, as well as ways to achieve them. Since every organization has a unique culture and norms, the attributes and approaches to exemplary practices are not prescriptive. However, there are some evidence-based approaches that can be applied in dissimilar ways to achieve similar outcomes. Lessons learned from experience, exemplars from Magnet institutions, and support from the literature offer directions and solutions that apply to a variety of practice settings and put an exemplary professional nursing practice within reach.

THE PROFESSIONAL PRACTICE MODEL— A PRIMARY COMPONENT

A nursing department's professional practice model (PPM) exists within the overall culture of a healthcare organization and must be aligned with it. The department's strategic vision, values, and priority initiatives should parallel the organization's mission, vision, and values. The professional practice model needs to include nursing's values, leadership, collaboration, professional development, and a care delivery system. Other components may be included in the professional practice model, but these key attributes must be included and addressed in the design and implementation.

Clarifying nursing department-specific strategy through the development of a PPM ensures that:
- Nurses are able to define and live by the principles and values that guide their practice.
- There are definitions, standards, and structures in place to guarantee that nurses ultimately control their own practice.
- Nurses interact with patients and families in a way that enhances their control and independence.
- Nurses interact with each other and with other disciplines in a collaborative and effective way.
- There are resources and systems in place to ensure competency, professional development, recognition, and rewards.
- There are systems for, and approaches to, performance management, career advancement, and peer review.
- There are structures in place for departmental decision-making and priority-setting (typically through a shared governance model).
- Nurses explicitly design or adopt a care delivery model or philosophy of patient care that guides their everyday practice. This usually can include but is not limited to:
  – Staffing standards
  – Assignments that ensure continuity of care
  – Skill mix
  – Communication standards within and across care settings
  – Educational requirements for nurses and others supporting nursing care
  – Novice-to-expert support systems
  – Competency models
- Nurses have identifiable mechanisms for monitoring and improving care, including needed resources such as technology, personnel, and education.

The components described here form the basis of a PPM as defined by Hoffart and Woods (1996), and Wolf and Greenhouse (2007). *See* Figure 6.1

Figure 6-1. Components of a Professional Practice Model

Generally, the attributes of an organization's PPM and the care delivery system within which it operates are drawn from an evidence-based theoretical framework such as the American

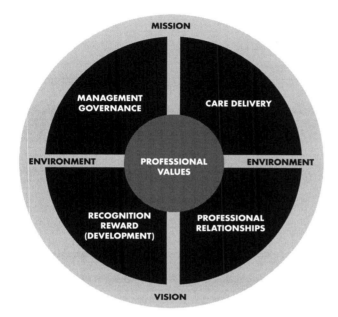

Source: Hoffart & Woods, 1996. Reprinted with permission.

Association of Critical-Care Nurses (AACN) Synergy Model, Watson's Caring Model, patient-centered care, relationship-based care, family-centered care, or primary nursing. The PPM uses standards and guidelines developed by professional associations such as a state's Nurse Practice Act, AACN Standards of Practice, American Nurses Association (ANA) Scope and Standards of Practice and Code of Ethics, Association of Operating Room Nurses (AORN) Standards of Practice, Oncology Nursing Society (ONS) Standards, American College of Obstetricians & Gynecologists (ACOG) Guidelines, and American Organization of Nurse Executives (AONE) Standards of Practice. The Magnet Model itself now forms the basis of many PPMs by incorporating the model's five major components (Transformational Leadership; Structural Empowerment; Exemplary Professional Practice; New Knowledge, Innovations and Improvements; and Empirical Outcomes), as well as the 14 Forces of Magnetism. Tiedman and Lookinland (2004) suggest care delivery models that evolve or become favorable within organizations and across disciplines are often based on the economic, political, and social issues of a given period.

To further explicate the elements of an exemplary professional practice, it is necessary to look closely at each element. These include:
• Frameworks for ensuring autonomy, accountability, and peer review
• Frameworks for ensuring and supporting competence and ethical practice

- Frameworks for ensuring privacy, security and confidentiality, workplace advocacy, and diversity
- Approaches to building a culture of safety
- Frameworks for interdisciplinary collaboration and leadership
- Methods for quality care monitoring and improvement

CARE DELIVERY SYSTEMS: PATIENT-, FAMILY-, AND NURSE-CENTERED

The care delivery system is integrated within the PPM. In Magnet hospitals, care delivery systems are patient- and family-centered, efficient, and collaborative.

Structural Components

The emergence of new care delivery models has opened the door to many additional innovations, specifically in the areas of nursing roles and nursing activities. Some examples of new nursing roles include: resource nurse, admission and discharge nurse, emergency department (ED) patient liaison, clinical nurse leader, patient navigator, stroke coordinator, lactation consultant, transition nurse, bariatric coordinator, quality outcomes nurse, infection control nurse, clinical documentation specialist, nurse recruiter, occupational health nurse, simulation educator, nurse ethicist, informatics nurse, and pain resource nurse. These innovations continue to highlight the importance of the professional nurse as coordinator of care. This coordination also extends to interdisciplinary relationships and nurse collaboration with advanced practice nurses (APNs).

The premises set forth in ANA's nurse staffing principles (ANA, 1999, 2005) lend support and guidance to the adoption of nurse staffing models that better meet the needs of patients and nurses. ANA advocates that staffing be based on enhancing patient outcomes and nurses' work–life balance. Successful organizations demonstrate the value of patient care assignments that provide continuity, match nurse competencies with patient needs, and quickly adjust to fluctuating workload and acuity. For example, many organizations use rapid response and stroke teams to meet patient needs during times of increased acuity. Others are investigating the feasibility of implementing acuity-adapted units.

Twelve-hour shifts, late-start shifts, self-scheduling, and closed floating are options explored by organizations on the Magnet journey. Some have instituted pilot programs designed by staff nurses to respond to patient needs in an increasingly complex healthcare system. Examples include team admissions and free charge roles. As organizations design their care delivery models, one inherent component is the manner in which assistive personnel will be incorporated. Delegation of and accountability for patient care is the sole responsibility of the professional nurse. As care models are developed and tested within organizations, metrics must be established to measure the effective use of personnel, as well as the patient's perspective of the quality of care received.

Process Components

Communication and information sharing have emerged as significant elements of the care delivery model. As consumers become more vocal in expressing their needs, patients and families are now at the center of many healthcare decisions. This, coupled with a nationwide focus on patient safety, has generated significant communication improvements such as walking rounds, shift huddles,

SBAR (Situation, Background, Assessment, Recommendation) communication frameworks and techniques, bedside shift reporting, patient care rounds, and pre-admission and post-discharge phone calls. Electronic medical records (EMR), telehealth medicine, and ever-more-sophisticated technology improve access to real-time information and enhance point-of-care decision-making.

As nursing departments align their strategic vision with the overall goals of their organizations, they scrutinize how patient care is delivered and determine which theoretical basis most appropriately defines nursing care. Some applications for Magnet status cite Watson's Theory of Human Caring, Kristen Swanson's Theory of Caring, Dorothea Orem's Theory of Self-Care, Katherine Kolcaba's Comfort Theory, Relationship-Based Care, AACN's Synergy Model, and Patricia Benner's From Novice to Expert Model.

Outcomes

Wolf and Greenhouse (2007) determined that care delivery outcomes are measured from the patient's, staff's, and organization's perspectives. Outcome variables include nurse-sensitive indicators, patient and staff satisfaction, turnover and vacancy rates, and financial measures. Outcome measurement must be continuous. One way to achieve this is through shared governance structures. By developing a robust shared governance program, care delivery outcomes can be evaluated at the unit level, across units, and at the department level. Unit-level evaluation allows for staff engagement and sustainability. Analysis can be accomplished using performance dashboards, report cards, and national databases. As part of the shared governance structure, outcome information is shared horizontally within councils. Another way for nurses to evaluate care delivery is the National Database of Nursing Quality Indicators® (NDNQI®) annual RN satisfaction survey, which monitors the professional practice environment and nurse perception of the quality of care delivered.

PROFESSIONAL PRACTICE MODEL EXEMPLAR

Mercy Medical Center in Baltimore, MD, used an interactive approach to develop a professional practice model that was then used to drive a nursing strategic plan. This plan was further developed at each of the unit levels, and the key areas that were addressed included leadership, culture, care delivery, collaborative practice, professional growth and development, evidence-based practice, research and innovation, and recruitment and retention. All of the key elements of a professional practice model were included, and others were added based on the needs of the organization. *See* Figures 6-2 and 6-3.

FRAMEWORKS FOR ENSURING AUTONOMY, ACCOUNTABILITY, AND PEER REVIEW

As MacDonald notes, professional autonomy indicates a "privilege of self-governance" that allows professionals substantial control over their practice with significant room to exercise their judgment (MacDonald, 2002). Nurses, like other professionals, are able to set and enforce standards of practice and have the right to exercise professional judgment according to those standards. Accountability for professional practice entails procedures and processes used by individuals and groups to justify and take responsibility for activities and actions. In health care, there is accountability to patients, professional organizations, and colleagues with a focus on competence and legal and ethical conduct, as well as development and adherence to professional standards. Professional associations, such as licensure boards, govern the practice of individual members (Emanuel & Emanuel, 1996).

Figure 6-2. Exemplar of a Professional Practice Model

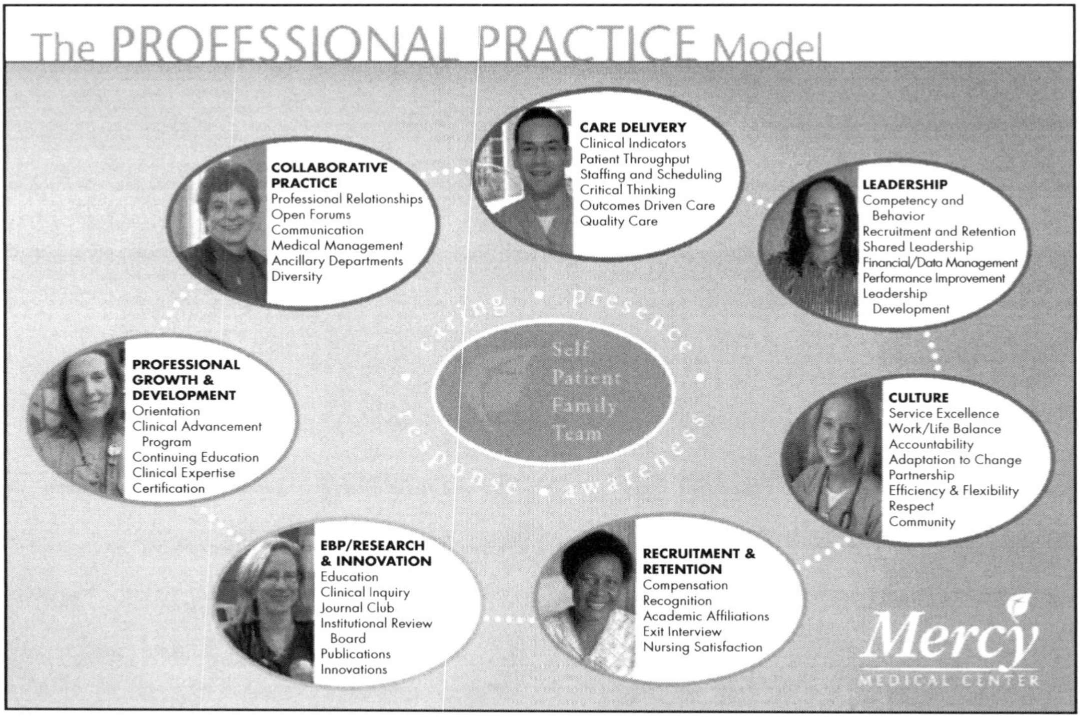

Source: Mercy Medical Center, Baltimore, MD. Reprinted with permission.

Figure 6-3. PPM Translated into the Nursing Strategic Plan

Nursing Division Vision Statement: To promote a culture of nursing and service excellence based on collaborative relationships, education, empowerment, evidence-based practice and research.

Leadership	Culture	Care Delivery	Professional Growth & Development	Recruitment & Retention	EBP/Research & Innovation	Collaborative Practice
Finance	Patient Satisfaction	Caring Model	Clinical Advancement Program	Vacancy	Technology	Bunting Tower Transition
Leadership Development	Service Excellence	Quality Improvement	Professional Development	Turnover	Evidence-Based Practice	Teamwork
Shared Governance	Community Outreach	Patient Safety	Peer Review	Nursing Satisfaction	Research	
	Magnet Status	Throughput				

Source: Mercy Medical Center, Baltimore, MD. Reprinted with permission.

Structural Components

Knowledge, information, and resources are available in the practice environment for care delivery decisions based on evidence and ethical principles, and in collaboration with other disciplines. A shared decision-making structure is in place so that nurses at all levels of the organization are involved and represented.

Process Components

When providing care, nurses have the authority and responsibility for clinical decision-making that directly impacts patient outcomes. Nurses are able to use their expertise for operational decision-making as well, such as the design of practice environments and staffing. Processes are in place for nurses to use performance and self-appraisal, including goal setting and peer review, on a routine basis.

Outcomes

When developing frameworks that ensure autonomy, accountability, and peer review, nurses have access to, and routinely use, current literature, professional standards, evidence, and data to support clinical decision-making and autonomous practice. In a state-wide study of New Jersey nurses' skills and access to evidence-based practice, for example, Cadmus et al. (2008) found that the use of computers and databases at Magnet hospitals differed significantly from non-Magnet facilities. Magnet participants sought information more often from a librarian, the Internet, conferences, or workshops; more of them identified, evaluated, utilized, and participated in research; and they rated the quality and availability of print, online, and other resources as adequate or more than adequate more often than in non-Magnet facilities.

In other Magnet settings, nurses have used performance appraisals and peer reviews for professional development and accountability. This allows them to initiate changes and make independent decisions in the practice environment.

Magnet organizations offer numerous examples of how nurse autonomy, accountability, and peer review can underscore the ability to utilize information and resources, make decisions, and resolve issues related to patient care or operational issues:
- Use professional practice guidelines as a basis for practice and practice changes.
- Practice within the scope of the profession while developing and implementing innovative solutions to common problems based on the latest evidence.
  - Use practice standards and specialty guidelines to make practice changes leading to improved care.
- Develop and use clinical ladder programs that allow direct care nurses to advance without leaving the bedside.
  - Use mentors or peer support to assist with professional development within the program.
  - Use councils or boards, with direct care nurse participation, to address promotions, salary increases, and disciplinary actions.
- Ensure access to information by means of the Internet and library:
  - Around-the-clock access to library materials, electronic articles and journals, research databases, e-books, images, videos, sounds, theses, and dissertations.
  - Library support staff.
  - In large organizations, this level of support is available on multiple campuses.

- Access literature and evidence at the point of care.
  - Computers are available in every patient room and nursing unit so nurses have access to online texts, professional journals, and professional nursing organizations' web sites to provide immediate responses to clinical questions and obtain supporting evidence.
- Use evidence to develop clinical practice guidelines to direct practice.
- Participate in unit-based councils where questions by staff nurses are discussed and lead to changes in practice.
- Staff nurses take action, advocate, and work collaboratively with physicians and other disciplines to achieve safe, patient- and family-centered, quality-driven, evidence-based patient outcomes.
- Conduct a variety of nurse-led clinics, with patient care education materials developed by staff nurses.
- Be involved in staffing and equipping new patient care areas.
- Performance appraisal incorporates peer review at all nursing levels across the organization.
- Direct care nurses use a professional portfolio for self-appraisal of professional development over time.

FRAMEWORKS FOR ENSURING AND SUPPORTING COMPETENCE AND ETHICAL PRACTICE

Professional competence has been defined by the Institute of Medicine (IOM) as the "habitual and judicious use of communication, knowledge, technical skills, clinical reasoning, emotions, values, and reflection in daily practice for the benefit of the individuals and community being served" (IOM, 2000). Such competence depends on and includes using clinical skills, scientific knowledge, and moral development; acquiring and using knowledge to solve problems; using biomedical psychosocial data in clinical reasoning; communicating effectively with patients and colleagues; and the willingness, patience, and emotional awareness to use these skills judiciously and humanely (Epstein & Hundert, 2002).

The ANA Code of Ethics for Nurses with Interpretive Statements (2001) contains nine provisions, which define the following eight values: safe, ethical, and competent care for patients or clients; the health and well-being of both the nurse and the patient; a patient's right of choice; dignity for the patient and the nurse; confidentiality of medical information; justice; accountability; and quality practice environments. These values provide a basis for ethical decision-making and professional practice (Lachman, 2009).

Structural Components

Information and ongoing professional development programs, in-services, and continuing education are available for staff and managers to continuously improve knowledge and expertise. Organizational support for competency-based skill development, clinical advancement, certification, and formal education is essential for building an educated and skilled nursing staff. To address complex ethical issues related to nursing practice and patient care, nurses need access to a variety of expert resources. Organizational policies and procedures are in place for the discussion and resolution of ethical and moral dilemmas and conflicts by interdisciplinary teams, committees, or panels.

Process Components

Access to leaders and managers for support is important for staff nurses to demonstrate their clinical expertise and be recognized (Laschinger, Almost, & Tuer-Hodes, 2003). Availability of experts, such as APNs, nurse educators, and external consultants offers ongoing opportunities to enhance clinical knowledge, skills, and decision-making. A code of ethics and the ability of nurses to seek assistance at the time moral or ethical situations are being confronted not only provide support but also enhance the delivery of care under difficult circumstances.

Examples of strategies used by Magnet organizations to support competent practice and manage complex ethical issues:

- Flexible scheduling and tuition assistance for education
- Ongoing continuing education and staff development sessions and courses
- Advanced practice nurses and nurse educators in clinical areas, often on all shifts for education, mentoring, and consult
- Financial assistance, workshops, and information for pursuit of certification
- Financial and staffing support for nurses to attend national, regional, and local conferences
- A well-developed, competency-based evaluation system, beginning with orientation
- Unit-based access to ethics resource information and guides, both written and electronic

- Ethics consults at any time, for any shift
- An active ethics committee that provides not only resources for consultations, but also the need for ongoing education and development of committee members and staff throughout the organization; through visibility and accessibility creates a climate that fosters open discussion of ethical concerns throughout the organization; and includes representatives from all disciplines
- External ethics experts available to the organization and the ethics committee for consultation and staff development
- Multidisciplinary ethics rounds that allow clinical caregivers the opportunity to discuss difficult emotional, social, or ethical issues that arise when caring for patients
- Annual Ethics Week and other events held throughout the year to address ethical issues
- Outreach to community groups

Outcomes

There are increased rates of certification and academic degrees for nurses at all levels of the organization. Evidence indicates nurses actively consult from both internal experts and external sources for clinical and ethical issues. Direct care nurses have positive perceptions of the support of the organization, nurse leaders, and managers for professional development and advancement, education and certification, and clinical skill and competency acquisition.

Magnet organizations support competent professional practice and deal with complex ethical situations by providing systems through a variety of strategies. (*See* Examples of Strategies.) One unique way a Magnet organization provides opportunities for nurses to develop new skills and knowledge is through temporary job exploration through re-assignment. For example, a nurse unit manager will be gone for an extended holiday or leave, and the position is posted as a temporary opening for which other nurses can apply. This strategy is used to determine if the nurse is right for the role, and to give more nurses greater responsibilities and better understanding of new positions and different units. These nurses are supported by nurse educators as they learn new skill sets and apply them in a protected time period, which can last up to 12 months.

FRAMEWORKS FOR ENSURING PRIVACY, SECURITY, CONFIDENTIALITY, WORKPLACE ADVOCACY, AND DIVERSITY

"Privacy, in the context of health information, refers to the ability of an individual to prevent certain disclosures of personal health information to any other person or entity. Confidentiality means the condition under which personal health information obtained or disclosed within a confidential relationship will not be redisclosed without the permission of the individual. Security is defined as the personal and electronic measures that grant access to personal health information" (Rothstein, 2007). These concepts are reflected in the Magnet Sources of Evidence.

Structural Components

In Magnet organizations, codes of ethics, policies, and procedures are in place that:
- Meet the healthcare needs of diverse patient populations;
- Provide a non-discriminatory environment for patients and staff;
- Identify and manage problems related to incompetent, unsafe, or unprofessional conduct;
- Provide for workplace advocacy; and
- Protect patient security, confidentiality, and privacy in the delivery of care, information technology, and research.

Process Components

Education is provided to enhance cultural competence and to ensure the proper use and protection of written and electronic confidential information. Processes and resources are available to identify and manage problems related to incompetent, unsafe, or unprofessional conduct. The organization, with nurse involvement, identifies and addresses disparities in the management of the healthcare needs of diverse patient populations and promotes a non-discriminatory climate for patients and staff.

Outcomes

Evidence shows that nurses use resources to meet the unique needs of patients and families, and that they are able to resolve issues related to patient privacy, security, and confidentiality. Organizational initiatives for workplace advocacy issues, such as caregiver stress, diversity, rights, and confidentiality are demonstrated.

Here are some examples of how Magnet organizations achieve results in these areas:
- Establish procedures for producing patient education materials in different languages, including development, translation, review, and evaluation.
- Provide interpreter services for the hearing-impaired or those with limited English proficiency.
- Offer multiple tools for non-English-speaking populations, including an Internet translator program to enhance cultural information and care, and a free repository for external use of patient education material in 17 languages.
- Establish interdisciplinary teams (with nurse members) with special training in cultural competency to help non-English-speaking patients, families, and visitors, or those with special needs.
- Increase staff awareness and understanding of different cultures and faith traditions in the patient population to ensure that varying dietary needs are met, and that interfaith services and events are offered.

- Train and develop staff working with individuals and families whose loved ones face serious illness or the end of life.
- Offer programs to increase the number of ethnically diverse student nurses and pair them with staff of similar ethnicity.
- Provide healthy environment options, such as healing gardens for staff and patients; an exercise facility; free conference facilities for professional and educational use; and areas for shift report, education, and renewal of the spirit.
- Provide organizational wellness programs for staff and family members that include health assessment, coaching, incentives, and "paybacks" that reduce insurance fees and premiums.
- In one long-term care facility, nurses adapted a model of care specific to their patient population. They formed "neighborhoods," with the same nurses, nursing assistants, and rehabilitation technicians assigned to the same patients on a continual basis. This model provides continuity, establishes a bond, and builds trust among patients, caregivers, and families.

APPROACHES TO BUILDING A CULTURE OF SAFETY

In the mid-1990s, following several highly publicized hospital errors (Conway et al., 2007; Reid-Ponte et al., 2003), the landmark work of the airline industry (Hamman, 2004; Thomas et al., 2004), and publication of IOM's compelling report *To Err is Human* (2000), patient safety came to the forefront. An evolving knowledge base and mounting evidence have emerged to drive creation of best practices to ensure cultures of safety in healthcare organizations. As part of the work of updating the Magnet Model in 2008 (Wolf et al., 2008), the expectation of advancing a safety culture within a Magnet hospital was added as a Source of Evidence.

Structural Components

There are several structural components necessary to ensure that a culture of safety is advancing in an organization. They start with a commitment from the board of trustees that safety is a priority. This is followed by written policies or standards. (*See* Patient Safety Examples.) Unit-based "safety champions" are common in healthcare organizations that prioritize safety. Safety champions receive advanced education to acquire and share quality and safety expertise and build unit-based imperatives that advance safety. In addition, there is a focus on workplace safety in areas such as needles, ergonomics, and infection control.

Examples of policies and standards in Magnet organizations that address patient safety:

- A fair and just culture (Connor et al., 2007)
- Sentinel events
- Root cause analysis
- Patient/family apology
- A patient safety officer
- Patient safety rounds

- Clinicians and staff at the "sharp edge of error" (Reason, 1990) have resources for coping and recovering
- Departments of quality and safety that formally organize error reporting
- Error mitigation approaches
- Inclusive committees of front-line staff, patients, and families
- Safety briefings
- Regular safety alerts or safety newsletters to communicate with staff about errors or near misses

Process Components

Safety cultures advance through a commitment to respect, collaboration, authenticity, transparency, diversity, and inclusion. This commitment starts at the top and must be consistently demonstrated by executive leadership. In the process of carrying out the structural elements of a safety culture described above, the behaviors of the senior team, managers, physicians, and nurses must be consistent with action orientation; active listening; accountability (versus blame); safety over convenience; integration of people and tasks; system thinking; process improvement; high regard for the knowledge worker; open and transparent sharing of information and perspective; building the reality of no fear of reprisal; and a commitment to interdisciplinary collaboration and partnering with patients and families to advance quality and safety. In organizations that advance a safety culture, leaders shoulder the burden of error. If the error was a result of system gaps, the error was essentially a responsibility of the organization and its leaders.

> **Boone Hospital Center (Columbia, MO) Exemplar**
> Patient safety is a key component of the organization's Quality Pillar. The narrative provided a number of exemplars that described patient safety activities and initiatives and the resources to support these activities. Staff throughout the organization were able to discuss their role in patient safety and it was clearly evident that this focus permeates the culture of the organization. Patient safety topics were evident in the work of numerous committees and in organizational communication tools such as bulletin boards and newsletters. For their work in patient safety, the organization has received the HealthGrades Distinguished Hospital Award for Patient Safety and has been recognized as a Best-Performing Hospital in Overall Patient Safety.

Outcomes

Organizations that prioritize and consistently advance their safety culture have mechanisms in place to measure its impact and determine that outcomes are commensurate with the safety goals. These include active monitoring of error reporting, surveying staff about their perceptions of a safety culture, and more general staff satisfaction surveys. Additionally, these organizations complete active error mitigation and formal risk assessment activities annually. They have human resource policies in place that ensure blame is not the first line of defense in examining and acting on errors, but rather system thinking and accountability. Commitment to a robust quality infrastructure and process improvement is demonstrated by a number of high-profile improvement projects selected annually, which focus on patient safety and impact executive compensation. (*See* Boone Hospital Center Exemplar.)

FRAMEWORKS FOR INTERDISCIPLINARY COLLABORATION AND LEADERSHIP

In Magnet hospitals the process of care delivery is interdisciplinary in nature. Care delivery teams are often composed of individuals prepared within a given discipline, each bringing a unique knowledge and skill set. Acknowledgment of the importance of interdisciplinary collaboration is one of the original Forces of Magnetism and was further advanced in the 2008 Magnet Model.

Structural Components

Care-giving teams don't function without effective leadership to set team norms, standards, and expectations. Interdisciplinary care teams can be hierarchical and unilateral in decision-making, or have shared leadership and collaborative decision-making. Experience shows that collaborative teams co-led by multiple disciplines (nurse–physician, physician–pharmacist, nurse–pharmacist, social worker–physician, etc.) are more likely to be effective, productive, and satisfied than teams that are hierarchical and unilateral. When such teams are led by two individuals with equal status, a truly collaborative group forms—one that is steeped in respect, equal contribution, diversity, and efficiency.

Process Components

Sharing and implementing ideas and expertise across disciplines enable a comprehensive approach to care delivery. Leading or participating in such teams requires a significant investment of commitment, time, and energy, but offers the potential for highly effective care (Cowan et al., 2006). Developing teams that work more effectively is now a priority in health care. Training is a common initiative in hospitals today, especially in operating rooms, delivery rooms, and emergency rooms. It is a growing practice in cardiology, oncology, and primary care (Mann et al., 2006). This work focuses on improved coordination, communication, and decision-making between team members and patients with the aim of improving outcomes.

Nationwide Children's Hospital (Columbus, OH) Exemplar

An exemplar of this organization's interdisciplinary work to address continuous quality and process improvements is the "One Team" value. This value is described in the organizational literature as "We are One Team":

- We collaborate across boundaries.
- We communicate openly.
- We routinely seek input from others.
- We leverage our diverse strengths.

This value is lived throughout the organization and was frequently mentioned by the nursing staff. A specific example that was highlighted during the site visit was the prevention of retinopathy of prematurity (ROP) in infants. A multidisciplinary team met and developed a process for identifying and ensuring that all neonates who met the criteria were screened at appropriate intervals; the parents were kept informed of the status of their infant; and follow-up interventions were scheduled. Significant outcomes have been achieved, and a new role for a nurse coordinator was established.

The Joint Commission (TJC) has prioritized various communication-improvement strategies including SBAR, hand-off procedures, and other approaches (TJC, 2010).

Outcomes

There is limited research evidence that supports the premise that effectively led, collaborative, interdisciplinary care teams improve patient care processes and outcomes (Boyle, 2004; Cowen, 2006; DeChairo-Marino, 2001; Grumbach, 2004; Horbar, 2004; Houldin, 2004). However, practice environment research supports the idea that the more collaborative and respectful team members perceive they are of each other, the higher quality of care they perceive they deliver (Aiken et al., 2002; Aiken et al., 2004; Friese et al., 2008). (*See* Nationwide Children's Hospital Exemplar.)

METHODS FOR QUALITY CARE MONITORING AND PROCESS IMPROVEMENT

The new Magnet Model has streamlined and advanced the commitment to quality monitoring, quality improvement, and clinical, patient-centered workforce, and organizational outcomes. Two of the original Forces of Magnetism focused on these structures and processes. They are now embedded into three of the five model components: Exemplary Professional Practice; New Knowledge, Innovations and Improvements; and Empirical Outcomes. Hence, an organization's commitment to quality continues to be the bedrock of excellence. Within the Exemplary Professional Practice component, the focus is on implementing the resources and processes to ensure quality patient care and continuous improvement.

Structural Components

Organizations that prioritize quality and process improvement invest in systems that continuously educate staff and leadership about the technology and best practices that support system thinking, lifelong learning, and quality improvement. Many of these organizations create processes for internal and external benchmarking of best practices, including the IHI (Institute for Healthcare Improvement), Lean, Toyota, ISO 9000, and PDSA (Plan, Do, Study, Act) models. Others create unique infrastructures that use priority settings, project and portfolio management, quality improvement (QI) project teams, and scorecards to advance their quality agenda. Many believe the Magnet Recognition Program® is a structure to ensure and advance quality.

Process Components

The Journey to Magnet Excellence™ serves as the benchmark for quality nursing practice and patient care. These standards provide an organization the structure to systematically evaluate nursing within the context of its specific culture. Evaluation of practice, then, is an essential structure and process to keep us informed about how we are doing. Effective mechanisms of measurement that evaluate the reliability of care processes are essential, as practices in a complex adaptive system can erode without our knowledge. Magnet requirements ensure that there is a system to identify and evaluate strengths as well as areas in need of improvement. The first step to improvement is building the capacity to know.

Outcomes

Outcome practices in nursing and medicine are subject to many influences: production pressures, autonomous practitioners, memory, fatigue, and experience, among other factors. Nurse-sensitive outcomes for inpatient services have been identified, and measurement systems to evaluate and benchmark them are now in place. Through national and statewide initiatives, such data are now transparent, helping patients decide where to receive care, and motivating nursing organizations to focus on improvement. It's important, therefore, that the data be valid and reliable. Ensuring that systems are in place to produce reliable data is itself an outcome. (*See* North Carolina Baptist Hospital of Wake Forest University Baptist Medical Center Exemplar.)

SUMMARY

In the future, many external forces will influence the changes required in professional practice models. Patients will continue to become more knowledgeable about managing both their health and their chronic disease states. The next generation of people needing care will be more technologically savvy, more engaged in their health needs, and more likely to be partners with their healthcare professionals. The way healthcare systems are organized will be changing rapidly in the next 10 years as reimbursement will be emphasized for more aspects of the continuum of care, rather than just an acute care episode of illness. Hospitals are going to be increasingly accountable for prevention of hospital-acquired events, and as a result new systems will be put in place to assure monitoring and evaluation of patients outside the hospital walls.

The knowledge available on the Internet will grow, as will the self-care movement, and the role of the nurse will continue to move to one of integrator, navigator, coach, and caregiver. The essential tenets of healing and caring will expand within the current medical model framework and will influence the values that nurses uniquely bring to the healthcare team. The need for compassion, caring, respect, and dignity will be the bedrock for the practice models created in the future. The public will increasingly call for validation of practitioner competency and expect a safe, highly reliable quality care experience. Creating a practice environment that promotes and ensures excellence requires a complex, dynamic set of structures and processes. Care delivery systems will need to be developed that are efficient, well-coordinated, nimble, and patient-centered. Nurse leaders will be called on to be creative in the development of these care delivery systems, and experimentation and evaluation will be increasingly important to determine which models are most effective. Through implementing these structures and processes, and evaluating the results, Magnet nurses will ensure a professional expert and excellent nursing practice that advances safe, high-quality patient- and family-centered care.

Hospital Exemplar: North Carolina Baptist Hospital of Wake Forest University Baptist Medical Center

The mechanisms for ensuring comprehensive dissemination of quality data to all stakeholders are substantial and of high quality, from the vision statements and structural entities responsible for quality data management to the standardized postable reports with explanatory footnotes visible in all patient care units. Numerous human and electronic resources are available to assist stakeholders in fully understanding processes and outcomes related to quality initiatives, including members of the house-wide Quality Council, members of the Compliance and Quality Team, APNs, and members of the Nursing Clinical Systems staff.

The appraisers verified the process by which pain management data are disseminated to all stakeholders in the organization. Evaluation occurs by a multidisciplinary Pain Committee led by a triad: an Oncology CNS, an MD, and an MD anesthesiologist. Data on satisfaction with pain management, assessment, and reassessment go to the Quality Council of Nursing Shared Governance and the unit manager. Mass e-mails are also cited as a method of sharing organizational data such as core measures. The Pain Committee provides an annual report to the Patient Safety Committee at the organizational level.

Additionally, the organization-wide Pain Committee established a Pain Management Subcommittee that involves approximately 40 direct care nurses who are supported by peers and managers to regularly attend the monthly 5:30–6:30 p.m. meetings. The groups have used the Failure Mode and Effects Analysis (FMEA) process to look at PCA incidents and have also established a web site that has an innovative dose calculator to support effective patient pain management by all providers.

REFERENCES

All URLs retrieved September 12, 2010.

Aiken, L., Clarke, S., Cheung, R., Sloane, D., & Silber, J. (2004). Relationship between patient mortality and nurses' level of education. *Journal of the American Medical Association, 291*(11), 1322–1323.

Aiken, L., Clarke, S., & Sloane, D. (2002). Hospital staffing, organization and quality of care: Cross-national findings. *International Journal for Quality in Healthcare, 14*(1), 5–13.

American Nurses Association. (1999). *ANA principles for nurse staffing*. Washington, DC: Author.

American Nurses Association. (2001). *Code of ethics for nurses, with interpretive statements*. Washington, DC: Author.

American Nurses Association. (2005). *Utilization guide for the ANA principles for nurse staffing*. Washington, DC: Author.

Boyle, D. K. & Kochinda, C. (2004). Enhancing collaborative communication of nurse and physician leadership in two intensive care units. *Journal of Nursing Administration, 34*(2), 60–70.

Cadmus, E., Van Wynen, E. A., Chamberlain, B., Steingall, P., Kilgallen, M. E., Holly, C., & Gallagher-Ford, L. (2008). Nurses' skill level and access to evidence-based practice. *Journal of Oncology Nursing Administration, 38*(11), 494–503.

Connor, M., Duncombe, D., Barclay, E., Bartel, S., Borden, C., Gross, E., Miller, C., & Reid-Ponte, P. (2007). Creating a fair and just culture: One institution's path towards organizational change. *Joint Commission Journal on Quality and Patient Safety, 33*(10), 617–624.

Conway, J., Nathan, D., Benz, E., Shulman, L., Sallan, S., Reid-Ponte, P., Bartel, S., Connor, M., Puhy, D., & Weingart, S. (2007). Key learning from the Dana-Farber Cancer Institute's ten-year patient safety journey. In *ASCO 2006 educational book*. Retrieved on September 12, 2010 from http://www.asco.org/ASCOv2/Education+%26+Training/Educational+Book?&vmview=edbk_category_edbooks_view&confID=40&category=Practice%20Mangement%20and%20Professional%20Issues

Cowan, M. J., Shapiro, M., Hays, R. D., Afifi, A., Vazirani, S., Ward, C. R. & Ettner, S. L. (2006). Ettner, S. L., et al. (2006). The effect of a multidisciplinary hospitalist/physician and advanced practice nurse collaboration on hospital costs. *Journal of Nursing Administration, 36*(2), 79–85.

DeChairo-Marino, A. E., Jordan-Marsh, M., Traiger, G., & Saulo, M. (2001). Nurse/physician collaboration: Action research and the lessons learned. *Journal of Nursing Administration, 31*(5), 223–232.

Emanuel, E. J., & Emanuel, L. L. (1996). What is accountability in health care? *Annals of Internal Medicine, 24*(2), 229–239.

Epstein, R. M., & Hundert, E. M. (2002). Defining and assessing professional competence. *Journal of the American Medical Association, 287*(2), 226-235.

Friese, C., Lake, E., Aiken, L., Silber, J., & Sochalski, J. (2008). Hospital nurse practice environments and outcomes for surgical oncology patients. *Health Services Research, 43*(4), 1145–1163.

Grumbach, K., & Bodenheimer, T. (2004). Can health care teams improve primary care practice? *Journal of the American Medical Association, 291*(10), 1246–1251.

Hamman, W. (2004). The complexity of team training: What have we learned from aviation and its application to medicine? *Quality and Safety in Health Care, 13*(Suppl 1), 72–79.

Hoffart, N., & Woods, C. (1996). Elements of a nursing professional practice model. *Journal of Professional Nursing, 12*(6), 354–364.

Horbar, J., Plsek, P., Leahy, K., & Ford, P. (2004). The Vermont Oxford network: Improving quality and safety through multidisciplinary collaboration. *NeoReviews, 5*(2), e42–e49.

Houldin, A. D., Naylor, M. D., & Haller, D. G. (2004). Physician-nurse collaboration in research in the 21st century. *Journal of Clinical Oncology, 22*(5), 774–776.

Institute of Medicine (IOM). (2000). *To err is human: Building a safer health system*. Washington, DC: National Academies Press.

The Joint Commission (TJC). (2010). *2010 national patient safety goals*. Retrieved from www. jointcommission.org/patientsafety/nationalpatientsafetygoals

Lachman, V. D. (2009). Ethics, law, and policy. Practical use of the nursing code of ethics: Part 1. *MEDSURG Nursing, 18*(1), 55–57.

Laschinger, H. K., Almost, J., & Tuer-Hodes, D. (2003). Workplace empowerment and Magnet hospital characteristics. *Journal of Nursing Administration, 33*(7/8), 410–422.

MacDonald, C. (2002). Nurse autonomy as relational. *Nursing Ethics, 9*(2), 194–201.

Mann, S., Marcus, R., & Sachs, B. (2006). Lessons learned from the cockpit: How team training can reduce errors in L&D. *Contemporary OB/GYN, 51*(1), 1–7.

Reason, J. (1990). *Human error*. Cambridge, England: Cambridge University Press.

Reid-Ponte, P., Conlin, G., Conway, J., Grant, S., Medeiros, C., Nies, J., Shulman, L., Branowicki, P., & Conley, K. (2003). Making patient-centered care come alive: Achieving full integration of the patient's perspective. *Journal of Nursing Administration, 33*(2), 82–90.

Rothstein, M. A. (2007). Health privacy in the electronic age. *Journal of Legal Medicine, 28(4)*, 487–501.

Thomas, E. J., Sexton, J. B., & Helmreich, R. L. (2004). Translating teamwork behaviors from aviation to healthcare: Development of behavioral marker for neonatal resuscitation. *Quality and Safety in Health Care, 13*(Suppl 1), 57–64.

Tiedeman, M. E., & Lookinland, S. (2004). Traditional models of care delivery, what have we learned? *Journal of Nursing Administration, 34*(6) 291–297.

Wolf, G., & Greenhouse, P. K. (2007). Blueprint for design, creating models that direct change. *Journal of Nursing Administration, 37*(9), 381–387.

Wolf, G., Triolo, P., & Reid-Ponte, P. (2008). Magnet Recognition Program: The next generation. *Journal of Nursing Administration, 38*(4), 200-204.

New Knowledge, Innovations, and Improvements

Mary Jo Assi, MS, RN, APRN-BC, AHN-BC
Deborah Zimmermann, DNP, RN, NEA-BC
Brenda Kelly, MA, RN, NEA-BC

Were there none who were discontented with what they have, the world would never reach anything better.
Florence Nightingale

It is essential to bridge the gaps between innovators, research, and the field.
Donald Berwick

INTRODUCTION

Advances in science and increases in patient complexity have accelerated the need for nurses with the skills and knowledge to manage a challenging and increasingly diverse healthcare environment. In the last century, the population over age 65 increased exponentially and by the year 2030, 20% of U.S. citizens will be over 65 and living with chronic illnesses requiring nursing care (Gavrilov & Heuveline, 2003, p. 2; SSDAN, 2010). As a profession, nursing has, in large part, transitioned from task-oriented to knowledge-based practice (Evans & Donnelly, 2006), and it is the expectation that Magnet® organizations will facilitate the completion of this transition. Nursing knowledge practiced from a systematic and evidence-based approach results in effective care and optimal patient outcomes (Kirkham, Baumbusch, Schultz, & Anderson, 2007; Melnyk, Fineout-Overholt, Stone, & Ackerman, 2000). An evidence-based approach supports high-quality care and provides a structure for critical and scientific analysis.

Magnet organizations consciously integrate evidence-based practice and, through research, drive new knowledge and innovation. The ability to innovate is critical to any organization's success; for a Magnet organization, such ability is by definition essential and necessary. Therefore, the Magnet environment supports risk taking, uncertainty, and failure as part of the journey to success. This chapter examines the fundamentals of evidence-based practice, research, and innovation, along with exemplars illustrating how organizations have actualized the Sources of Evidence in a variety of settings.

DEFINITION OF TERMS

The terms commonly used in the translation of new knowledge and scientific practice are described here using the agreed-upon definitions from the most recent Magnet manual (ANCC, 2008).

Evidence-Based Practice

"The conscientious use and integration of the best research evidence with clinical expertise and patient preferences in nursing practice (adapted from Sackett et al., 2000). Evidence-based practice is a science-to-service model of engagement of critical thinking to apply research-based evidence within the context of patient values to deliver quality, cost-sensitive care. It is distinguished from practice-based evidence, a practice-to-science model in which data are derived from interventions thought to be effective but for which empirical evidence is lacking. Providers are engaged in data collection, analysis, and synthesis to inform practice" (ANCC, 2008, p. 2).

Nursing Research

At the time of publication, the 2008 Magnet manual included a definition of nursing research from Polit and Hungler (1995) as "a systematic search for knowledge about issues of importance to the nursing profession" (ANCC, 2008, p. 63). Polit and Beck (2010) have expanded the definition to "systematic inquiry that uses disciplined methods to answer questions to solve problems. The ultimate goal of research is to develop, refine, and expand a body of knowledge" (p. 4).

Quality Improvement and Performance Improvement

"Systematic data-guided activities designed to bring about immediate improvement in healthcare delivery in particular settings (Lynn et al., 2007, p. 667)" (ANCC, 2008, p. 64).

Innovation

"Innovation in service delivery and organization [is] a novel set of behaviors, routines, and ways of working that are directed at improving health outcomes, administrative efficiency, cost effectiveness, or users' experience and that are implemented by planned and coordinated actions (Greenhalgh, 2004, emphasis added)" (ANCC, 2008, p. 62).

Performance Improvement vs. Research

A common difficulty for organizations on the Magnet journey is the differentiation between performance improvement and research. In performance improvement, clinicians use the evidence from existing research, guidelines, or data to enhance professional practice and organizational performance when a response to an immediate problem is needed. Research uses a scientific process to generate new knowledge to answer unresolved questions of importance to professional nursing practice.

When First Health of North Carolina established a goal to reduce tobacco use in their community, they implemented the national guidelines set forth by the Centers for Disease Control and Prevention. They used the evidence, combined with innovative approaches, to achieve performance improvement. When the evidence is not available or does not satisfy the needs of the reviewers, scientific methods of research are necessary to determine how to achieve the best outcomes. When nurses working in an endoscopy unit in Rochester, New York, could not find guidelines on post-procedure positioning, the nurses enlisted the assistance of a researcher to help them develop a research study. The nurse scientist guided the nurses in refining their study question, in developing a hypothesis and research design, and finally in obtaining approval from their human subjects review board. After the study was completed, the nurses changed their practice based on findings, and they disseminated study results at a regional professional nurses symposium.

In summary, performance improvement is the process of implementing current scientific evidence to drive change. Research adds to the knowledge of nursing for the purpose of improving patient outcomes. Performance improvement and research are foundational to the science of nursing and guide us in our pursuit to answer the question "How can we do this differently to produce a better outcome?" Both research and performance improvement can involve innovation. The following exemplar illustrates an innovation in driving performance improvement.

> *Penny Blake, MS, RN, a director of nursing at Brenner Children's Hospital of Wake Forest University Baptist Medical Center in Winston-Salem, NC, recognized the value of capturing incident information of near-misses. She observed that staff were consistently reporting actual incidents, but were inconsistently reporting incidents that were caught and resolved before they reached the patient.*
>
> *She engaged her staff in an evaluation of the reporting process and together they developed a program called Great Catch. The objectives were for staff to identify and document near-misses and errors in the hospital's patient safety net reporting database and receive recognition for the "great catches." The reports were evaluated for process failures and actions were taken to correct these and prevent future errors. Over an 11-month period, reports of incidents increased by 50%, while actual errors decreased by 18%. The proactive approach to identify near-misses and reward staff for reporting them resulted in significant overall improvement.*

THE CASE FOR EVIDENCE-BASED PRACTICE

Just as Magnet recognition is identified as the gold standard for nursing excellence, evidence-based practice is arguably the gold standard for care delivery. Nurses are central to the process of developing evidence, and by doing so they demonstrate the contribution of nursing to achieving improved patient outcomes. Benchmark databases are available for comparison of outcomes with a wide range of similar institutions, and nurse-sensitive indicators are now used to evaluate the overall quality of care that nurses provide.

Medicare's identification of *never events* and refusal to reimburse healthcare organizations for additional care related to these occurrences have brought traditionally nursing issues into the boardroom. Never before have the subtleties of skin assessment or the shearing forces of patient positioning in the operating room been discussed with such fervor and passion as they are today. Because never events are nurse-sensitive and directly related to nursing care, a new focus on the value, role, and contribution of nursing is emerging nationwide. Therefore, it is nursing's responsibility to ensure that current science is used in practice.

CORE VALUES FOR EVIDENCE-BASED PRACTICE AND RESEARCH

Knowing what questions to ask, where to find answers, and then using that empirical evidence in clinical care is key to professional nursing. If asked, nurses would respond that they support evidence-based practice, yet successful institutionalization of a culture of inquiry that ensures best practice for every patient is a challenge and not universally accomplished. How does a nurse manager create and maintain a culture that inspires a nurse balancing multiple patient care issues to go to the literature for answers at 2 a.m.? Or bring forward a compelling question for research at the close of a busy shift?

Clinical leaders must promote an environment of lifelong learning and inspire a commitment to a vision of the preferred future (Leach, 2005, p. 228). It is the responsibility of nursing leaders to encourage questioning and insist that bedside nursing practice be based on the latest science. Melnyk et al. (2004) found that when nurses are provided comprehensive education, mentorship, and access to Internet databases, evidence-based practice is accelerated. Subscriptions to major journals and up-to-date texts are insufficient for consistent implementation of evidence-based care. When leaders establish a standard requiring that every policy, pathway, and protocol—at every level—be based on the latest science, expectations are set and demonstrate the organization's commitment to a core value: evidence-based practice. Nothing is more rewarding to a nurse leader than to hear staff debate a clinical issue or unit-based policy and challenge each other to cite a source of information.

ESTABLISHING A CULTURE OF INQUIRY

Questioning the status quo and thriving in an environment of uncertainty take leadership and sustained commitment to action. Melnyk and Fineout-Overholt (2005, pp. 28–29) suggested regular prompting of clinical questions using a structured format in forums of everyday practice. Assisting nurses to pose well-formed questions enhances communication and instills the confidence to embark on research. When there is insufficient evidence to support practice, there is opportunity to design and conduct research.

Most nurses fear they do not have sufficient expertise to conduct research, even though some of the best ideas and studies come from routine clinical situations. Potential research questions arise from practice every day. For example, how can humor be used therapeutically to reduce pain levels in post-operative surgical patients? What are the primary patient indicators that result in an ICU-to-floor nurse consultation and subsequent transfer to the intensive care unit? What medical unit physical design results in a reduction of nosocomial infection rates?

Unfortunately, conflicting priorities often cause research questions to lie dormant and unanswered. One key to moving from idea to study is linking staff and doctorally prepared nursing scientists. A formal arrangement between a college and a healthcare organization, or the creation of a team linking staff nurses, advanced practice nurses (APNs), and researchers from different specialties, coupled with clear expectations from leaders on how research is to be conducted, will fertilize the ground for ongoing nursing scholarship as evidenced by the following exemplar.

> *Amy E. Winecoff, BSN, RN, COHN-S, the nursing director of employee health at Lake Norman Regional Medical Center (LNRMC) in Mooresville, NC, recounts her beginning interest in nursing research (in McLaughlin & Bulla, 2010). She describes her fear and lack of confidence to take those first necessary steps to develop a research study. She talked to a colleague at the local university who supported her idea and assigned a master's-educated nursing student to help her get started. She also received support from the LNRMC Nursing Research Council, which gave her the confidence to take the first step.*

> *Amy revamped the procedures and processes associated with the management of employee back injuries. LNRMC implemented a one-on-one class on safe back mechanics for every new employee. The class is taught by a physical therapist and is repeated for an employee if a back injury occurs. One year after implementation, annual lost work days were reduced from 5.6 to 1.1, and the average cost of a back injury decreased from $2,266 to $364. Amy's advice to anyone thinking about research: "just do it" (McLaughlin & Bulla, 2010, p. 272).*

Nursing standards, protocols, and pathways must be based on science. A passionately vigilant attention to evidence-based practice is required until it is hardwired and encultured in the nurses. When practice issues arise in rounds, staff meetings, or shared governance forums, evidence must be the basis for decision-making. Establish expectations and accountability for scientific practice in job descriptions, clinical advancement programs, and performance appraisals. Advancement of a research agenda and utilization of evidence-based practice are enhanced by designating evidence-based practice champions on units to operationalize the vision, the plan, and a commitment to a culture of inquiry. Systems and processes need to be in place to create the space where these issues can be identified and moved into the sphere of evidence-based practice and research.

Key to the successful creation of a culture of evidence-based practice is the allocation of clinical information and resource availability at all times. With these resources comes the need for education. Organizations have instituted toolkits, journal clubs, brown-bag seminars, and hotlines dedicated to evidence-based practice. These strategies promote a safe environment for nurses to ask questions and discuss practice issues.

The Institute of Medicine (2004) and nurse researchers have suggested that improving the healthcare system will enhance patient safety and achieve better patient outcomes (Aiken, Clark, Cheung, Sloane, & Silber, 2003; Estabrooks, Midozi, Cummings, Ricker, & Giovannetti, 2005; Tourangeau et al., 2006). Because registered nurses constitute the majority of the healthcare workforce, it is logical that promoting research that fills the gap in scientific practice will improve patient outcomes. Thus, Magnet hospitals serve as leaders in furthering the development of new knowledge and innovation in goal-oriented, formalized research programs.

ESTABLISHING AN EVIDENCE-BASED PRACTICE INFRASTRUCTURE

How do nurse leaders proceed from the concept of evidence-based practice and nursing research to robust organizational enculturation? Dedicated support from nursing leadership is an essential first step to creating the foundation for a successful program (Funk, Champagne, Tornquist, & Wiese, 1995; Retsas, 2000; Titler & Everett, 2006). Formulating a vision and a conceptual framework congruent with existing organizational values and structure helps guide the process in the early stages, and then sustains and expands the program as it develops (Drenkard, 2005; Hockenberry, Walaen, Brown, & Barrera, 2007).

A useful method in determining organizational capacity for research is to conduct a readiness assessment. The knowledge gained can help determine current barriers, strengths, and weaknesses to evaluate the state of an existing program, or assist in development of a new research program uniquely tailored to meet the needs of a specific organization. The Evidence-Based Practice Beliefs Scale and Evidence-Based Practice Implementation Scale (Melnyk, Fineout-Overholt, & Mays, 2008), the Barriers Scale (Funk, Champagne, Wiese, & Tornquist, 1991), or the Research Involvement Survey, Nursing Research Attitude Scale, and the Research Environment Scale (Smirnoff, Ramirez, Kooplimae, Gibney & McEvoy, 2007) are all existing tools that an organization may find valuable.

BUILDING NURSING RESEARCH CAPACITY

When a clear picture of organizational readiness and capacity is determined, the next step is creation of infrastructure to support and sustain a hospital-based nursing research and evidence-based practice program. The structure should be designed to meet the needs of an organization and take into account organizational and nursing goals, mission, values, vision, and philosophy, and align with both the nursing theoretical framework and the professional practice model. There is no one best model, and the nursing literature abounds with examples from outstanding organizations such as Massachusetts General Hospital (Larkin, Cierpial, Stack, Morrison, & Griffith, 2008) and Texas Children's Hospital (Hockenberry et al., 2007) that can provide a starting point to stimulate discussion and ideas in other organizations.

As the conduct of nursing research requires higher levels of academic preparation and experience, nursing research committees and activities may tend to operate apart from the overall governance framework. To avoid this type of drift and promote a truly integrated program, delineation of structure must firmly establish nursing research and evidence-based practice within the governance framework and include nurses at all levels of the organization (Gawlinski, 2008; Titler & Everett, 2006). During initial planning, consideration of appropriate roles for nurses with varied educational preparation and thoughtful inclusion of education and training in the conduct of nursing research for all staff are useful to ensure that direct care nurses have the opportunity to participate in nursing research beyond the data collection phase (McCloskey, 2008). In the following exemplar, one Magnet organization formalized mentorship and funding of nurse scientists.

In 2005, University of Rochester Medical Center–Strong Memorial Hospital in Rochester, NY, developed a year-long, federally funded research internship experience for nursing staff, leadership, and APNs. The program exposes nurses to research and evidence-based practice principles and provides mentors to help them complete a project relevant to their area of practice. Selected participants receive one paid day per month to attend formal education sessions. The depth and quality of the curriculum, as well as the number of interns trained and outcomes reported, provide an exemplary and innovative framework to engage nurses at all levels of the organization. The hospital also established the Center for Innovation and Clinical Advancement (CICA) to link clinical information technology to clinical practice through expert change agents. CICA has since evolved as the driving force that enculturates research and evidence-based practice at Strong Memorial Hospital.

SUSTAINED OPERATIONAL LEADERSHIP

The core leadership group for nursing research within a healthcare organization should include an expert as an active participant in development and implementation of all activities (ANCC, 2008, p. 22). This relationship may vary depending on the structure the organization chooses as a best fit. It may involve a formal or informal partnership with an academic institution, or obtaining the services of a doctorate-prepared nurse scientist either as a consultant or through permanent employment. However, to facilitate this critical relationship, at least one nurse research expert must be involved in strategic planning and goal setting in order to build nursing research capacity and provide coaching and mentorship to novice researchers (Fineout-Overholt, Levin, & Melnyk, 2004). Ongoing decision-making for nursing research and evidence-based practice activities in an organization is strengthened by ensuring that staff nurses who are both qualified and available to participate in research activities are allotted sufficient time away from direct patient care for this important work. This group should include advanced practice nurses and educators because their educational preparation and roles are uniquely suited to development of, and participation in, nursing research and evidence-based practice programs (Malloch & Porter-O'Grady, 2010, p. 73; Melnyk & Fineout-Overholt, 2005, p. 216). Questions and issues important to nursing occur at the point of practice and form the basis for original research within the organization. Care should be taken to ensure that people from all levels of nursing, including management, are core participants in the research and evidence-based practice decision-making body. Creating a separate budget line for nursing research and evidence-based practice further underscores ongoing support from nursing leadership. Both fiscal and human resources are required to create the structure to implement, sustain, and expand a program of nursing research over time. A dedicated budget for research and evidence-based practice helps nurse leaders prioritize structural components needed to move the nursing research agenda forward. Depending on the current status of a particular nursing research program, monies may be used for a variety of activities. (*See* Resources for Evidence-Based Practice Programs.)

Resources for Evidence-Based Practice Programs

- A doctorally prepared nurse consultant or employee
- Staff time to participate in nursing research committee or council work
- Internal and external education for staff on research and evidence-based practice topics of interest to the organization
- Implementation of a nurse research fellow or training program for direct-care nursing staff, APNs, and nurse leaders
- An annual nursing research seminar or similar venue to highlight nursing research specific to the organization
- Improving electronic access for staff to evidence-based practice and nursing research-related literature and other tools such as SPSS data analysis software
- Access to a statistician to assist with data analysis
- Creation of a multi-hospital nursing research and evidence-based practice consortium

TRANSLATING NEW KNOWLEDGE INTO PRACTICE

Translating new knowledge into practice is challenging, particularly in complex organizations such as hospitals. Evidence-based practice conceptual models may provide a template and a standardized process for moving findings from research and national guidelines into practice. A model provides a standardized template for clarifying a clinical or practice problem, reviewing the literature, critically assessing research, identifying practice changes, implementing change, and finally evaluating processes and outcomes across an organization.

Selection of an existing evidence-based practice model may facilitate the implementation of a framework for hardwiring research utilization and evidence-based practice within an organization. Gawlinski and Rutledge (2008) published a practical guide for healthcare organizations that outlines the steps in selecting a model. Melnyk and Fineout-Overholt (2005, pp. 196–204) reviewed several contemporary organizational frameworks, including IOWA, Advancing Research and Clinical Practice through Close Collaboration (ARCC), Kitson, and Rosswurm and Larrabee models. Another example, Disciplined Clinical Inquiry (DCI), is described as "unique" by Malloch and Porter-O'Grady (2010, p. 35) in that the clinician's perspective is foundational to the model's design. On the other hand, an organization may decide to adapt or create its own model to meet specific needs. Whatever the choice, a methodical, formal approach to clinical inquiry, research, and translation of evidence-based practice into daily nursing practice is critical for Magnet designation and to advance nursing science within a healthcare organization.

The requirements for meeting the Magnet Sources of Evidence do not recommend or support one specific model over another. More important is that the selected model fit the organization and that staff are adequately prepared to describe it and use it in practice. This is accomplished in a number of ways, including educational sessions on evidence-based practice, toolkits provided to nursing units or departments, and clinical nursing rounds. Organizations with an established process often incorporate it in orientation, with education-focused reviews and updates as appropriate to ensure that all levels of nursing are apprised of current activities.

COMMUNICATION AND DISSEMINATION OF ACTIVITIES

The impact of evidence-based practice and nursing research activities is proportional to the degree to which new knowledge is communicated to nurses at all levels in the organization. If, for example, staff nurses identify a clinical issue, research the issue, and conclude that a change in practice is warranted, how is such information consistently disseminated to ensure best practice and outcomes in all areas of the system? While creating a sound infrastructure for a nursing research and evidence-based practice committee or council is an essential step, organizations may fall short if the work accomplished is not readily accessible or communicated to clinicians (Fineout-Overholt, Melnyk, & Schultz, 2005; Oermann, Roop, Nordstrom, Galvin, & Floyd, 2007).

The structures that support nursing research and evidence-based practice should include elements that specifically address both vertical and horizontal communication of committee or council-based activities to ensure full dissemination (Gawlinski, 2008; Newhouse, Dearholt, Poe, Pugh, & White, 2007). Inclusion of dissemination methods in the charter, or in a graphic representation that demonstrates the relationship between formal organization-wide structures such as nursing practice, nursing leadership, performance improvement, and nursing research, and that extends to the unit level, is a good way to accomplish this. Creative implementation of information technology has many applications to inform best practice. Weaver, Warren, and Delaney (2005) provide two compelling examples of technology-based innovations to disseminate evidence-based practice principles and information: 1) the transition from paper-based protocols to the clinical information system allowing bedside nurses immediate access to evidence-based data specific to individual patient care needs, and 2) a successful collaboration between the University of Kansas School of Nursing and Cerner Corporation to develop a sophisticated, computer-based education program to embed principles of evidence-based nursing practice in the baccalaureate nursing curriculum.

Whatever methods are adopted to advance nursing research and evidence-based practice in an organization, the goal is that nurses at all levels are able to "connect the dots." In Magnet organizations, there is a clear expectation that nurses can articulate nursing research and evidence-based practice initiatives with respect to their professional role within the organization, particularly when current information and knowledge recommend that change is warranted. Structure and process should support translation of new knowledge into the practice arena, as well as rigorous monitoring and data analysis to evaluate the impact of change (outcomes) at the point of practice.

MEASURING OUTCOMES

Nursing makes an essential contribution to patient, nursing workforce, organizational, and consumer outcomes. "The empirical measurement of quality outcomes related to nursing leadership and clinical practice in Magnet organizations is imperative" (ANCC, 2008, p. 52). A conceptual framework that promotes effective structure and process to advance nursing research and evidence-based practice is a powerful tool to foster and facilitate nursing practice changes based on current science. It also provides organizational consistency in the translation of new knowledge into practice. The incorporation of empirical outcomes as the fifth component of the 2008 Magnet Model marks a significant shift from previous models that emphasized structure and process as evidence of clinical quality and excellence. While these elements are the foundation for a successful program of research and evidence-based practice, the addition of measurable outcomes that meet pre-defined standards of excellence ensures accountability that structure and process are truly hitting the mark to improve nursing practice.

DISSEMINATION TO THE NURSING COMMUNITY

"Magnet organizations are expected to serve as mentors and lead the way in the provision of quality patient care and the creation of environments that contribute to the well-being of the workforce and the community at large" (ANCC, 2008, p. 34). A hallmark of Magnet organizations is a commitment to promote scientific inquiry through nursing research and evidence-based practice to expand the body of nursing knowledge and strengthen the science of nursing practice. While the evidence-based practice movement continues to gain momentum, significant obstacles are consistently reported in the literature, including lag between awareness of new knowledge and its translation into the practice arena (Fineout-Overholt, Melnyk, & Schultz, 2005).

Melnyk, Fineout-Overholt, Stetler, and Allan (2005) and others (Fineout-Overholt et al., 2005; Malloch & Porter-O'Grady, 2010, p. 27) suggest that one factor necessary to facilitate rapid advancement of evidence-based practice and research is a methodical approach to ensure wider dissemination of outcomes to the nursing community at large. At the organizational level, it is vital that nursing leadership create an environment that encourages, supports, and mentors nurses to share research findings and best practices internally and externally, through poster or podium presentations and publication (Broom & Tillbury, 2007). Leaders also should pursue opportunities to champion and participate in web-based technology and programs such as learning communities. Evolving technology offers an excellent platform to share new knowledge in a timely manner to promote rapid adoption of best nursing practices.

INNOVATION AT ALL LEVELS

Innovation is vital to the health and growth of all organizations (Kelley & Littman, 2005; Porter-O'Grady, 2008). This is particularly true in the current climate, where healthcare organizations are continually challenged to improve clinical practice and financial performance. The status quo ultimately fosters stagnation and complacency. A paradigm that encourages exploration of new and creative ideas, and encourages nurses at all levels to challenge the status quo is, in fact, what is really needed.

In Magnet hospitals innovative nursing practice occurs at all levels of nursing professionals, from the direct care nurse to the chief nursing officer (CNO). It encompasses the staff nurse who adapts a clinical practice to meet the needs of an individual patient and finds that the adaptation produces a positive outcome that can be applied to other patient care situations. It includes the manager who, based on careful analysis of unit-based data and root cause analysis related to falls, proposes a new staff role to enhance clinical quality and safety on the unit.

Organizations steeped in tradition, cautious, and inclined to wait and see when presented with new ideas are not well positioned to maintain the pace, much less lead the way, in today's complex and rapidly changing healthcare arena. In contrast, organizations that intentionally create an environment in which innovation is cultivated and embedded as a cultural norm in day-to-day operations have tremendous potential to shape the future of health care through consistent application of new and innovative quality practices. Innovative risk taking, including acceptance of the accompanying occasional failure, must be embraced by the executive leadership team as a strategic priority (Hughes, 2006; Newhouse, 2007).

Ultimately, the degree of success for any structured approach to innovation rests with leadership. In a study conducted by McMurray and Williams (2004), only 5% of nurse managers surveyed believed they possessed the skills and organizational support needed to be innovative leaders. This finding suggests that mentorship by executive nurse leaders related to innovation and innovative practice needs to be integral to the manager role. It is essential that executive nurse leaders clearly communicate that risk-taking is encouraged and that mistakes are sometimes inevitable and accepted as part of the process (Viney & Rivers, 2007). In Magnet organizations, there is a sense of adventure. Managers create an environment to engage and encourage direct-care staff to apply evidence-based innovative ideas and solutions to clinical and practice issues.

Innovations in Nursing Practice

Innovation is purposeful, science-based, and the result of a great deal of perspiration. One example was a program evaluation study conducted by clinical nurse specialist Sue Nickoley, RN, MS, GCNS-BC, and nursing leader Vicky Orto, MS, RN, NEA-BC, in their study of the impact of education and program changes in the care of seniors.

The purpose of their evaluation and their pre-test/post-test design was to determine the quality and effectiveness of a comprehensive geriatric program, using the national NICHE (Nurses Improving Care for Healthsystem Elders) program's evidence-based best practices. The researchers questioned whether proposed interventions would make a difference in the quality of geriatric nursing care within the organization. Their interventional strategy included implementation of a geriatric Age Matters! standard in patient care interventions and institution of a geriatric resource nurse (GRN) program. The GRN model of care included a GRN core course, GRN biweekly meetings, GRN practice rounds, GRN competency validation, a certification review process, and clinical practice changes. Outcome measures included pre- and post-intervention testing of staff nurses using the Geriatric Institutional Assessment Profile (GIAP) survey and the Geriatric Competencies for RNs in Hospitals. The results indicated unit-based experts in geriatrics in combination with standards of care for patients over 65 resulted in improved outcomes in geriatric knowledge, confidence, and an age-sensitive geriatric care environment compared to national benchmarks. The results were shared with staff within the organization and presented at the Twelfth Annual ANCC National Magnet Conference® in 2008. (*See* Innovative Partnership Exemplar.)

Innovative Partnership Exemplar: The Atlanta Veterans Administration

In Decatur, GA, the Atlanta Veterans Administration Medical Center faced challenges caring for veterans who had served in the military in Operation Enduring Freedom and Operation Iraqi Freedom. For the first time, large-scale services were needed for women veterans, as well as an overwhelming number of personnel discharged with significant physical and mental disabilities.

The nurses in this Magnet organization rose to the occasion, enhancing services for female veterans and for the home telehealth program. Other programs and clinics were initiated or enhanced specifically to help soldiers with complex physical and mental disabilities acclimate to civilian life.

INNOVATIVE PARTNERSHIPS

Magnet and Magnet-aspiring organizations recognize that innovation is a crucial element for growth, and that cutting-edge nursing practice is essential to provide the best possible patient care. Innovative partnerships with community-based entities, professional organizations, quality healthcare forums, and academic institutions provide organizations with incredible opportunities to promote innovative nursing practice in the healthcare arena. Without question, such partnerships can benefit both entities when mutual goals are clearly defined (Jeffs et al., 2006; Horns et al., 2007).

Reasons to create partnerships run the gamut. A CNO may choose to partner with an organization such as the American Nurses Association at the state or national level to create a workgroup to explore best practices to improve safe patient handling . Numerous organizations have benefited from partnerships with quality organizations such as the Institute for Healthcare Improvement (IHI) to participate in initiatives that improve practice and outcomes. Innovative partnerships between healthcare organizations and community-based programs and institutions can provide a platform to meet the needs of both on a number of levels. The decision to partner with local or regional community groups to provide focused support for vulnerable populations may in turn favorably impact utilization of healthcare dollars. Working with local high schools to engage students in programs designed to increase awareness of career opportunities in health care can be an effective means for recruitment.

Working across associations and organizations, Magnet hospitals have formed consortiums with their state nursing associations and other professional organizations to gather for best-practice sharing and research dissemination.

One example is the Virginia Magnet Consortium, which shares resources between the Virginia Magnet hospitals and the Virginia Nurses Association. Comprised of fifteen facilities, the Consortium meets regularly for networking and sharing their collective experiences to promote excellence in practice, and operates according to its mission statement: "The Virginia Magnet Consortium exists to unify our efforts to foster nursing excellence in the Commonwealth by building upon our collective Magnet experience." (Virginia Nurses Association, 2009)

Similar partnerships are forming in other regions such as New York State.

Innovative Partnerships for Education and Research

A question commonly raised by Magnet-aspiring organizations is, "Do all hospitals have to meet the same standards and Sources of Evidence related to research and evidence-based practice?" The question comes from community hospitals without academic affiliations, those with fewer beds in rural settings, and those in the international sector. The answer is yes, the same standards apply to all healthcare organizations for Magnet designation or re-designation. Since the inception of the Magnet Recognition Program, organizations from every sector have successfully met or exceeded goals related to nursing research and evidence-based practice. The partnerships, affiliations and creative resource sharing that occur in rural settings are strategies that these organizations have used to raise the level of participation in research activities and evidence-based practice. Some of the innovations have come in response to finding ways to raise the bar in these areas.

Hoyt (2006) describes a number of factors that may limit research and evidence-based practice utilization and dissemination in developing countries. These include wide disparities in education, limited access to continuing education, and severe shortages of healthcare personnel in certain regions of the world. To address this issue, the Dreyfus Health Foundation's "Problem Solving for Better Health" program was initiated in 2002 to provide a cost-effective, grassroots approach to educating and engaging nurses in 15 countries on four continents (Dreyfus Health Foundation, 2002). At last report, more than 3,500 nurses have initiated 2,200 projects aimed at improving the quality of health care in local communities (Smith, Hoyt, & Fitzpatrick, 2010). Despite obstacles, nurses have overcome what first seemed insurmountable barriers to find workable solutions. In a survey of 21 nurse administrators from community hospitals, participants ranked research as the least important attribute of the professional growth domain (Newhouse & Mills, 2001). Although the financial and human resource challenges in community and rural hospitals are significant, the CNO must establish the standard for evidence-based practice and nursing research. Nurse research must be one of the highest-ranked domains. Nurses in small hospitals assume great responsibility, and are frequently called upon to translate new knowledge into practice. (*See* Innovation in Partnerships: Clinical Partnership Program.)

In considering innovative solutions, partnerships can be pivotal in helping Magnet-aspiring organizations to achieve the goal of designation. One of the first steps is to ask nurses from Magnet hospitals for help. Magnet nurses love to mentor colleagues on the journey and are only waiting to be asked to serve. Another solution that has worked for many Magnet organizations is partnering with academia to build a robust program for research and evidence-based practice. Examples of how rural, small, and international organizations can link with academic institutions abound in the literature (Burns, Dudjak, & Greenhouse, 2009; Turkel, Ferket, Reidinger, & Beatty, 2008). Partnerships that truly benefit all stakeholders, such as the Clinical Partnership Program created between a community hospital in northern New Jersey and a local school of nursing, illustrate the power of this "win-win" scenario.

Innovation in Partnerships: Clinical Partnership Program: The Valley Hospital, Ridgewood, NJ

Innovative partnerships with academic institutions are often instrumental to the success of a research and evidence-based program agenda (Drenkard, 2005; Jamison, Fish, & Frandsen, 2009). In 2004, Linda Lewis, the CNO of a 451-bed Magnet-designated community hospital in northern New Jersey, and Dr. Kathleen Burke, the dean of nursing at the Ramapo College of New Jersey, created an innovative design for a clinical partnership. Hospital-based APNs serve as clinical associate faculty for students during on-site clinical rotations through completion of their BSN program. Student nurses have the opportunity to integrate Magnet values into their blossoming professional practice, and are mentored by APNs who are both content experts and familiar with all facets of nursing practice in the organization. The synergy created for continual exchange of ideas between clinical practice and academia enhances both. From the CNO's perspective, this partnership has created a pipeline to recruit new nurses who, upon graduation, are already very familiar with the organization. In addition, Dr. Burke serves as a consultant to the Valley Hospital for nursing research and evidence-based practice. In that capacity, she attends all Nursing Research Council meetings, provides mentorship to novice nurse researchers, and educates all levels of staff on research-related topics, and has been instrumental in working with the Nursing Research Council and nursing leadership to develop the annual strategic plan for advancement of nursing research within the organization.

Capturing Innovative Ideas

At the organizational level, Magnet hospitals must demonstrate the capacity to develop strategies that support and cultivate innovation, and describe the best practices and outcomes that result from the implementation of new and innovative ideas (ANCC, 2008, p. 32). The astute healthcare leader recognizes that innovation and the flexibility to respond to both internal and external forces in a timely and thoughtful manner are crucial to ensure best practices and outcomes for patient care (Donaldson & Rutledge, 1998; Porter-O'Grady & Malloch, 2010, p. 38). There is discussion among all segments of the profession to seek innovative solutions to immediate and long-term issues and challenges. Forums for networking and discussion related to innovative nursing practice are found on numerous professional and other health care-related web sites such as the AHRQ Innovations Exchange (http://www.innovations.ahrq.gov), IHI's Learning and Innovation Communities (http://www.ihi.org/IHI/Programs/Collaboratives), and the International Council of Nurses Innovations Database (http://www.icn.ch/innovations). The American Academy of Nursing cultivates nominations for "Edge Runners" that exemplify innovative nursing solutions to address healthcare delivery issues or the unmet health needs of specific populations (Weber, 2009).

Given that innovation is essential to moving nursing practice forward, it would stand to reason that organizations that systematically harness and implement innovative practices from all corners will excel in promoting and developing exemplary nursing practice. For this reason, the integration of structure and process to both recognize and capture innovative nursing practice at all levels on an ongoing basis is a goal that organizations may want to pursue (Greenhalgh, Robert, Macfarlane, Bate, & Kyriakidou, 2004; Porter-O'Grady, 2008; Price, 2006; Schumacher, Drenkard & Tornabeni, 2004).

One approach may involve intentionally and specifically including recognition of innovation in the shared decision-making structure. This could be accomplished by creating a committee or group charged with identifying and evaluating innovative ideas or recently implemented practices that have resulted in positive outcomes throughout patient care services. Another approach could be to include "innovative practice" as a standing agenda item in all staff, council, and committee meetings where nursing practice is routinely discussed. Asking, "Has anyone attended a conference, journal club, or network group this past month?" both highlights the expectation of shared learning and opens the door to capturing innovative ideas on a consistent basis. Whatever methods an organization chooses, the capacity to methodically capture great ideas and evaluate new best practices in a timely manner with an eye toward system-wide implementation is a worthy goal.

Magnet organizations serve as the fount of knowledge and expertise in the delivery of nursing care globally. Because nurses and the interdisciplinary teams within these healthcare organizations are solidly grounded in core Magnet principles, there is continual cultivation of a culture of inquiry and innovation. The best outcomes are achieved when nurses practice evidence-based care (Melnyk, 2002; Melnyk & Fineout-Overholt, 2005).

SUMMARY

Nurses in Magnet organizations are leading the reformation of health care and the profession. Their dedication to lifelong learning, research, and fastidious use of current science translates into organizational performance. Because of their unrelenting commitment, these organizations are improving the delivery of care and health outcomes in their patients, families, and communities. In Magnet organizations, structures are in place to facilitate finding solutions, and the answers are within reach. In Magnet organizations, the seemingly impossible is possible and is happening now.

Looking ahead, it is clear that breakthrough medical advances are coming at increasing speed. Creating a culture of innovation and sharing of new knowledge will be the necessary foundation if our patients are going to be able to receive the most advanced level of care possible. Undoubtedly, advances in technology and communication methodologies will be a key part of these innovations. The role of the nurse will remain closest to the patient, so the interpretation, integration, and coordination of this knowledge explosion will remain a core element of nursing practice. Along with research and innovation in patient needs for education, self-care management, management of chronic diseases, and the shift to wellness and prevention, the essential connection to the patient and the human caring interactions will be areas that nursing research will continue to develop as the future of health care unfolds. Magnet organizations are leading the way and embracing the future with eagerness.

REFERENCES

All URLs retrieved September 12, 2010.

Agency for Healthcare Research and Quality (AHRQ). (2010). AHRQ Innovations Exchange. Retrieved from http://www.innovations.ahrq.gov/index.aspx

Aiken, L. H., Clarke, S. P., Cheung, R. B., Sloane, D. M., & Silber, J. H. (2003). Educational levels of hospital nurses and surgical patient mortality. *Journal of the American Medical Association, 290*(12), 1617–1623.

American Nurses Credentialing Center. (2008). *Application manual: Magnet Recognition Program.* Silver Spring, MD: Author.

Broom, C., & Tilbury, M. (2007). Magnet status: A journey, not a destination. *Journal of Nursing Care Quality, 22*(2), 113–118.

Burns, H., Dudjak, L., & Greenhouse, P. (2009). Building an evidence-based practice infrastructure and culture: A model for rural and community hospitals. *Journal of Nursing Administration, 39*(7–8), 321–325.

Donaldson, N. & Rutledge, D. (1998). Expediting the harvest and transfer of knowledge for practice in nursing: Catalyst for a journal. *Online Journal of Clinical Innovations, 1*(2), 1–25. Retrieved from http://nurseweb.ucsf.edu/conf/cripc/knowart.pdf

Drenkard, K. (2005). Sustaining Magnet: Keeping the forces alive. *Nursing Administration Quarterly, 29*(3), 214–222.

Estabrooks, C. A., Midodzi, W. K., Cummings, G. G., Ricker, K. L., & Giovannetti, P. (2005). The impact of hospital nursing characteristics on 30-day mortality. *Nursing Research, 54*(2), 74–84.

Evans, R. J. & Donnelly, G. W. (2006). A model to describe the relationship between knowledge, skill, and judgment in nursing practice. *Nursing Forum, 41*(4), 150–157.

Fineout-Overholt, E., Levin, R., & Melnyk, B. (2004). Strategies for advancing evidence-based practice in clinical settings. *Journal of the New York State Nurses Association, 35*(2), 28–32.

Fineout-Overholt, E., Melnyk, B., & Schultz, A. (2005). Transforming health care from the inside out: Advancing evidence-based practice in the 21st century. *Journal of Professional Nursing, 21*(6), 335–344.

Funk, S., Champagne, M., Tornquist, E., & Wiese, R. (1995). Administrators' views on barriers to research utilization. *Applied Nursing Research, 8*(1), 44–49.

Funk, S., Champagne, M., Wiese, R., & Tornquist, E. (1991). BARRIERS: The barriers to research utilization scale. *Applied Nursing Research, 4*(1), 39–45.

Gavrilov, L., & Heuveline, P. (2003). *Aging of population.* Retrieved from http://longevity-science.org/Population_aging.htm

Gawlinski, A. (2008). The power of clinical nursing research: Engage clinicians, improve patients' lives, and forge a professional legacy. *American Journal of Critical Care, 17*(4), 315–327.

Gawlinski, A., & Rutledge, D. (2008). Selecting a model for evidence-based practice changes: A practical approach. *AACN Advanced Critical Care, 19*(3), 291–300.

Greenhalgh, T., Robert, G., Macfarlane, F., Bate, P., & Kyriakidou, O. (2004). Diffusion of innovations in service organizations: Systematic review and recommendations. *Milbank Quarterly, 82*(4), 581–629.

Hockenberry, M., Walden, M., Brown, T., & Barrera, P. (2007). Creating an evidence-based practice environment: One hospital's journey. *Journal of Nursing Care Quality, 22*(3), 222–233.

Horns, P., Czaplijski, T., Engelke, M., Marshburn, D., McAuliffe, M., & Baker, S. (2007). Leading through collaboration: A regional academic/service partnership that works. *Nursing Outlook, 55*(2), 74–78.

Hoyt, P. (2006). Problem-solving for better health nursing: A working approach to the development and dissemination of applied research in developing countries. *Applied Nursing Research, 19*(2), 110–112.

Hughes, F. (2006). Nurses at the forefront of innovation. *International Nursing Review, 53*(2), 94–101.

Institute for Healthcare Improvement (IHI). (2010). *Collaborative learning.* Retrieved from http://www.ihi.org/IHI/Programs/Collaboratives

Institute of Medicine (IOM). (2004). *Keeping patients safe: Transforming the work environment of nurses.* Washington, DC: National Academies Press.

International Council of Nurses (ICN). 2010. *Innovations database.* Retrieved from http://www.icn.ch/projects/Innovations-Database/

Jamison, P. A., Fish, A., & Frandsen, G. (2010, in press). Nursing Student Research Assistant Program: A strategy to enhance nursing research capacity building in a Magnet-status pediatric hospital. *Applied Nursing Research.* Posted on-line October 15, 2009

Jeffs, L., Affonso, D., MacMillan, K., Mathews, S., Bookey-Basset, S., Campbell, H., & Merkley, J. (2006). Building capacity for nursing research. *Canadian Nurse, 102*(8), 30–32.

Kelley, T., & Littman, J. (2005). *The ten faces of innovation: IDEO's strategies for beating the devil's advocate and driving creativity throughout your organization.* New York, NY: Currency/Doubleday.

Kirkham, S. H., Baumbusch, J. I., Schultz, A. S., & Anderson, J. M. (2007). Knowledge development and evidence-based practice: Insights and opportunities from a post-colonial feminist perspective for transformative nursing practice. *Advances in Nursing Science, 30*(1), 26–40.

Larkin, M., Cierpial, C., Stack, J., Morrison, V., & Griffith, C. (2008). Empowerment theory in action: The wisdom of collaborative governance. *Online Journal of Issues in Nursing, 13*(2). Retrieved from http://www.nursingworld.org/MainMenuCategories/ANAMarketplace/ANAPeriodicals/OJIN/TableofContents/vol132008/No2May08/ArticlePreviousTopic/EmpowermentTheory.aspx

Leach, L. S. (2005). Nurse executive transformational leadership and organizational commitment. *Journal of Nursing Administration, 35*(5), 228–237.

Lynn, J., Baily, M. A., Bottrell, M., Jennings, B., Levine, R., Davidoff, F., et al. (2007). The ethics of using quality improvement methods in health care. *Annals of Internal Medicine, 146*(9), 666–673.

Malloch, K., & Porter-O'Grady, T. (2010). *Introduction to evidence-based practice in nursing and health care* (2nd ed.). Sudbury, MA: Jones and Bartlett.

McCloskey, D. (2008). Nurses' perceptions of research utilization in a corporate healthcare system. *Journal of Nursing Scholarship, 40*(1), 39–45.

McLaughlin, M. M. K., & Bulla, S. A. (2010). *Real stories of nursing research: The quest for Magnet recognition.* Sudbury, MA: Jones and Bartlett.

McMurray, A., & Williams, L. (2004). Factors impacting on nurse managers' ability to be innovative in a decentralized management structure. *Journal of Nursing Management, 12*(5), 348–353.

Melnyk, B. M. (2002). Strategies for overcoming barriers in implementing evidence-based practice. *Pediatric Nursing, 28*(2), 159–161.

Melnyk, B. M., & Fineout-Overholt, E. (2005). *Evidence-based practice in nursing and health care: A guide to best practice.* Philadelphia, PA: Wolters Kluwer Health/Lippincott, Williams & Wilkins.

Melnyk, B. M., Fineout-Overholt, E., Feinstein, N. F., Li, H., Small, H. L., Wilcox, L., & Kraus, R. (2004). Nurses' perceived knowledge, beliefs, skills, and needs regarding evidence-based practice: Implications for accelerating the paradigm shift. *Worldviews on Evidence-Based Nursing, 1*(3), 185–193.

Melnyk, B. M., Fineout-Overholt, E., & Mays, M. (2008). The evidence-based practice beliefs and implementation scales: Psychometric properties of two new instruments. *Worldviews on Evidence-Based Nursing, 5*(4), 208–216. Erratum in *Worldviews on Evidence-Based Nursing, 6*(1), 49.

Melnyk, B. M., Fineout-Overholt, E., Stetler, C., & Allan, J. (2005). Outcomes and implementation strategies from the first U.S. evidence-based practice leadership summit. *Worldviews on Evidence-Based Nursing, 2*(3), 113–121.

Melnyk, B. M., Fineout-Overholt, E., Stone, P., & Ackerman, M. (1999). Evidence-based practice: The past, the present, and the recommendations for the millennium. *Pediatric Nursing, 26*(1), 77–80.

Newhouse, R. (2007). Creating infrastructure supportive of evidence-based nursing practice: Leadership strategies. *Worldviews on Evidence-Based Nursing, 4*(1), 21–29.

Newhouse, R., Dearholt, S., Poe, S., Pugh, L., & White, K. (2007). Organizational change strategies for evidence-based practice. *Journal of Nursing Administration, 37*(12), 552–557.

Newhouse, R., & Mills, M. (2001). Research in the community hospital. *Journal of Nursing Administration, 31*(12), 583–587.

Oermann, M., Roop, J., Nordstrom, C., Galvin, E., & Floyd, J. (2007). Effectiveness of an intervention for disseminating Cochrane Reviews to nurses. *MEDSURG Nursing, 16*(6), 373–377.

Polit, D. F., & Beck, C. T. (2010). *Essentials of nursing research: Appraising evidence for nursing practice.* Philadelphia, PA: Wolters Kluwer Health/Lippincott Williams & Wilkins.

Polit, D. F., & Hungler, B. (1995). *Nursing research: Principles and methods.* Philadelphia, PA: Wolters Kluwer Health/Lippincott Williams & Wilkins.

Porter-O'Grady, T. (2008). Creating an innovative nursing organization. *Voice of Nursing Leadership, 6*(2), 6–7. Retrieved from http://www.aone.org/aone/pubs/Voice/March2008Voice.pdf

Porter-O'Grady, T., & Malloch, K. (2010). *Innovation leadership: Creating the landscape of health care.* Sudbury, MA: Jones and Bartlett.

Price, B. (2006). Strategies to explore innovation in nursing practice. *Nursing Standard, 21*(9), 48–55, 58, 60.

Retsas, A. (2000). Barriers to using research evidence in nursing practice. *Journal of Advanced Nursing, 31*(3), 599–606.

Sackett, D. L, Straus, S. E., Richardson, W. S., Rosenberg, W., & Haynes, R. B. (2000). *Evidence-based medicine: How to practice and teach EBM* (2nd ed.). Edinburgh, Scotland: Churchill Livingstone.

Schumacher, E., Drenkard, K., & Tornabeni, J. (2004). Care delivery innovation in an integrated health system. *Nurse Leader, 2*(1), 52–55.

Smirnoff, M., Ramirez, M., Kooplimae, L., Gibney, M., & McEvoy, M. (2007). Nurses' attitudes toward nursing research at a metropolitan medical center. *Applied Nursing Research, 20*(1), 24–31.

Smith, B., Hoyt, P., & Fitzpatrick, J. J. (2010). *Problem solving for better health: A global perspective.* New York, NY: Springer Publishing Co.

Social Science Data Analysis Network (SSDAN). (2010). *Disability status of the aged.* Retrieved from http://www.censusscope.org/us/print_chart_aged_disability.html

Titler, M., & Everett, L. (2006). Evidence-based nursing: Sustain an infrastructure to support evidence-based practice. *Nursing Management, 37*(9), 14–16.

Tourangeau, A. E., Doran, D. M., Hall, L. M., Pallas, L. O., Pringle, D., Tu, J. V., & Cranley, L. A. (2006). Impact of hospital nursing care on 30-day mortality for acute medical patients. *Journal of Advanced Nursing, 57*(1), 32–44.

Turkel, M., Ferket, K., Reidinger, G., & Beatty, D. (2008). Building a nursing research fellowship in a community hospital. *Nursing Economic$, 26*(1), 26–34.

Viney, M., & Rivers, N. (2007). Front-line managers lead an innovative improvement model. *Nursing Management, 38*(6), 10, 14.

Virginia Nurses Association, Virginia Magnet Consortium. Accessed at http://www.virginianurses.com/displaycommon.cfm?an=1&subarticlenbr=94

Weaver, C., Warren, J., & Delaney, C. (2005). Bedside, classroom and bench: Collaborative strategies to generate evidence-based knowledge for nursing practice. *International Journal of Medical Informatics, 74*(11–12), 989–999.

Weber, D. O. (2009). Nursing innovations. *Hospital & Health Networks.* Retrieved from http://www.hhnmag.com/hhnmag_app/jsp/articledisplay.jsp?dcrpath=HHNMAG/Article/data/01JAN2009/090113HHN_Online_Weber&domain=HHNMAG

8

Empirical Outcomes

Rosemary Luquire, PhD, RN, NEA-BC, FAAN
Margaret Strong, MSN, RN, NE-BC

I think one's feelings waste themselves in words; they ought all to be distilled into actions which bring results.
Florence Nightingale

It is not possible to learn without measuring, but it is possible—and very wasteful—to measure without learning.
Donald Berwick

INTRODUCTION

A profession may have many characteristics, including a distinct body of knowledge; a basis in one or more undergirding disciplines from which it builds its own applied knowledge and skills; being organized into one or more professional associations; agreed-upon performance standards for admission to the profession and for continuance within it; a protracted preparation program, usually in a professional school on a college or university campus; a high level of public trust and confidence in the profession and in individual practitioners; a commitment to ongoing competence; and authority to practice through licensure, regulation, and credentialing (Kizlik, 2010).

A profession, such as nursing, is also marked by its continued ability to make a positive impact on society. Over the last 15 years, demand has grown for increased accountability and improved value from our country's healthcare system. Medical costs have soared, yet we have lower life expectancy and higher infant mortality rates than many other industrialized nations. Magnet® organizations are expected to create structures and implement and stabilize evidence-based processes that lead to improved outcomes for patients, the nursing workforce, organizations, and communities. Characteristically, Magnet organizations are never content with the status quo and constantly strive to improve their results. These organizations continually benchmark both internally and externally to identify best practices and opportunities for improvement. This chapter examines the history of the outcomes movement, the types of outcomes that are crucial for the highly accountable nursing organization to impact, and the responsibility of the nurse leader and direct-care nurse in driving improvement. It includes details about national benchmarking and variance analysis. In the wake of the increased demand for value-based health care, it explores the role of Magnet organizations to mentor and lead other healthcare providers in delivering optimal health outcomes in a cost-efficient manner.

HISTORY OF THE OUTCOMES MOVEMENT

Since the mid-1990s, the emphasis on outcomes reporting has gathered momentum thanks to work by organizations such as the National Quality Forum, the Joint Commission, and the Centers for Medicare and Medicaid Services(CMS). However, outcomes measurement and a focus on quantitative and qualitative results date back more than 150 years. They were introduced in 1855 by Florence Nightingale (1820–1910), who earned considerable attention for her mathematical and analytic work that measured post-operative complications, as well as her scheme for uniform hospital statistics. Nightingale's work led to a huge reduction in mortality rates in the Crimean War—from 42% to just 2.2% (Kopf, 1916). She also pioneered the use of pie charts and other easy-to-understand statistical graphics in her presentations. She is credited with introducing statistics to drive process improvement through the use of legitimate and meaningful data interpretation (Spiegelhalter, 1999; Nightingale, 1863). Her work was foundational in the creation of the first recognized nursing curriculum.

Subsequently, Ernest Codman (1869–1940), an orthopedic surgeon whose lifelong pursuit was to track patient care outcomes and identify opportunities for process improvement, became known as the founder of outcome management and evidence-based practice. Dr. Codman championed the "End Results Idea"—the common-sense notion that every hospital follow every patient long enough to determine whether treatment was successful. Otherwise, how could such failures be prevented in the future? Dr. Codman created the first morbidity and mortality conferences at Harvard University, which caused great angst among healthcare professionals. He insisted that results be made public so that patients could make informed decisions when choosing physicians and hospitals (Berwick, 1989). Dr. Codman was the first healthcare practitioner known to promote not only measurement but also data transparency to practitioners and the public. His vision went unrealized for 60 years until institutions finally began to create quality and financial scorecards (Donabedian, 1989; Neuhasuer, 1990). Even then, practitioners were hesitant to share results. It wasn't until the Institute of Medicine (IOM) released *To Err is Human: Building a Safer Health System* in 2000 that impetus built for closer evaluation and redesign of the healthcare system, with a greater focus on measurement and transparency (IOM, 2000).

The report generated fear and disbelief across the United States as the IOM reported that hospital errors contributed to as many as 98,000 deaths annually, and the cost of preventable adverse events ran as high as $29 billion. The report galvanized a call to action to improve the U.S. healthcare system; the status quo would not be tolerated. The IOM urged external organizations to find ways to make errors so costly that hospitals would be compelled to improve safety. CMS responded by implementing financial penalties for adverse events. The following year, IOM published *Crossing the Quality Chasm, A New Health System for the 21st Century*, which called for a focus on quality indicators to ensure that health care was based on the best available scientific knowledge (IOM, 2001). IOM required that care be safe, effective, patient-centered, timely, efficient, and equitable. Magnet hospitals have historically focused on improvement in many, if not all, of these dimensions.

As the Magnet Model has evolved, the Commission on Magnet (COM) and its constituents have put greater emphasis on Magnet hospitals' ability to show specific outcomes that reflect advanced knowledge and changing national imperatives. The Sources of Evidence published in 2008 require that hospitals demonstrate structures and processes that lead to exemplary outcomes (ANCC, 2008). These outcomes are reflective of the impact of bedside nurse leaders and nursing executives on patient and community outcomes, as well as nurse and organizational outcomes. Examples are outlined in Table 8-1.

Table 8-1. Examples of Empirical Outcomes

Patient Outcomes

Risk-adjusted mortality index
Healthcare-acquired infections
Falls and injuries associated with falls
Hospital-acquired pressure ulcers
Patient satisfaction
Patient perception of safety
Specialty population-specific outcomes

Nurse Outcomes

Level of nurse engagement
Level of nurse satisfaction
Nurse autonomy
Turnover and vacancy rates
Percentage of RNs with certification
Educational preparation of staff
Staff injury rates
Staff perception of work environment
Effectiveness of educational programs

Organizational Outcomes

Efficiency and/or elimination of wastes
Chief nursing officer impact on system-level change

Consumer Outcomes

Impact of community outreach programs
Community health and welfare

Source: ANCC, 2008.

When delineating expected outcomes, the COM did not simply adopt nurse-sensitive indicators from organizations such as the National Quality Forum or IOM. However, the convergence of these quality imperatives clearly influenced the Commission's work.

Table 8-2, a crosswalk between the IOM's six aims and Magnet Sources of Evidence, illustrates this convergence. Many professional practice or conceptual models (such as the Synergy Model) create an expectation for environments or structures that promote safe patient passage. Within this framework, the prevention of adverse events is foremost. Magnet institutions have made great strides in the application of evidence-based practices in clinical, educational, and leadership arenas. The impetus for delivering evidence-based strategies to promote patient well-being and staff expertise provides an effective and efficient way to ascertain desired results. Magnet hospitals must be able to demonstrate excellent clinical outcomes, as well as ensure that patients' perception of care reflects excellence in human caring and compassion. Magnet's focus on patients' perception of care is clearly congruent with IOM's emphasis on patient-centered care. Magnet also recognizes the clear correlation between staff engagement and work environment on patients' perception of care, length of stay, and complication rates.

As the Magnet Model was transformed, opportunities arose to harvest feedback and input from key stakeholders at national meetings. Nurse executives requested that specific outcomes be measured that reflected improvements in quality and efficiency. Their message was clear: Continue to drive waste out of the system through more efficient processes that would improve access to care and enhance the work environment. Nurse leaders also requested measurement of return on investment as resources were reallocated in operating or capital budgets. Stakeholders viewed this measurement as an assessment of nurse leaders' financial acumen, as well as their ability to effectively and efficiently influence resource allocation. While the Sources of Evidence do not specifically require documentation of outcomes that demonstrate equitable care (an IOM aim), Magnet hospitals are expected to understand patient and staff demographics and provide an environment that meets the unique needs of both.

BENCHMARKING

As IOM's six aims for improvement have become more embedded in bedside practices, nurses must have accurate data to make decisions about improvement opportunities and best practices. Benchmarking, an integral part of the ongoing quality improvement process, is one way to accomplish this. Healthcare organizations use two types of benchmarking: external and internal. External benchmarking shows data that affect care pillars, which include quality, finance, service, and people. An example is patient satisfaction. Patients at different healthcare organizations are asked the same questions and their answers are compared. The institutions can evaluate issues such as pain control, staff friendliness, and physician responsiveness. If a hospital consistently scores in the 95th percentile in one of these areas, a best practice is present and needs to be shared.

Internal benchmarking compares data among similar units within the organization, for example, patient falls data on all the medical and surgical units. The unit that scores consistently above the 95th percentile for the least number of falls probably has a best practice, which would be shared with the other units. As the information is incorporated into patient care plans, falls should decrease on all units.

Table 8-2. Institute of Medicine Aims and Magnet Sources of Evidence Crosswalk

Six Aims for Improvement (Institute of Medicine[1])	Magnet Sources of Evidence[2]
Safe	Application of the professional practice model. (*Exemplary Professional Practice*) Workplace safety improvements for nurses. (*Exemplary Professional Practice*) Nurse-sensitive indicators outperform national norms in the area of patient safety (*Exemplary Professional Practice*) Facility approach to error reduction. (*Exemplary Professional Practice*)
Effective	Outcome of strategic planning focused on improving system effectiveness. (*Transformational Leadership*) Preparation of workforce to better serve patients evidenced by improvement rates in number of nurses with formal education and professional certification. (*Structural Empowerment*) Effectiveness of continuing education programs. (*Structural Empowerment*) Application of evidenced-based practices and translation of knowledge into practice. (*New Knowledge, Innovations & Improvements*)
Patient-Centered	Application of the professional practice model in collaboration (client-centered) or communication with the patient and family. (*Exemplary Professional Practice*) Patient satisfaction data outperforms national norms in the areas of pain, education, courtesy, respect, and attentiveness to patient needs. (*Exemplary Professional Practice*) Staff satisfaction or engagement outperform national norms. (*Exemplary Professional Practice*)
Timeliness	Response time or access to care. (*Exemplary Professional Practice*)
Efficiency	Outcome of strategic planning focused on improved system efficiencies. (*Transformational Leadership*) Quality improvements realized based on specific allocation or reallocation of resources. (*Exemplary Professional Practice*) Improvement in practice related to technology and space design. (*New Knowledge, Innovations & Improvements*)
Equity	Results of community outreach programs. (*Structural Empowerment*) Outcomes of programs focused on the healthcare needs of diverse populations. (*Exemplary Professional Practice*)

[1]IOM, 2001, *Crossing the Quality Chasm.*
[2]ANCC, 2008, *Application Manual: Magnet Recognition Program*, pp. 25-33.

In 1994, the American Nurses Association (ANA) began its Safety and Quality initiative to explore and identify empirical linkages between nursing care and patient outcomes (www.nursingquality.org). The initiative led to the development and maintenance of the National Database of Nursing Quality Indicators® (NDNQI®). The indicators are nurse-sensitive, which reflect the structure, process, and outcomes of nursing care. Structure is indicated by nursing hours per patient-day, staff skill level, and the education and percentage of board-certified nurses. In the Magnet Model, Structural Empowerment includes these as Sources of Evidence. Process indicators measure assessment and intervention, as well as RN job satisfaction. In the Magnet Model, Exemplary Professional Practice includes these as Sources of Evidence. Outcomes that are nurse-sensitive are those that improve with greater quantity or quality of nursing care. Nurse-sensitive indicators are reflected in Empirical Outcomes in the Magnet Model. NDNQI's mission is to "aid the nursing provider in patient safety and quality improvement efforts by providing research-based national comparative data on nursing care and the relationship to patient outcomes."

NDNQI is the only national nursing quality measurement program that provides hospitals with unit-level reports for nurse-sensitive outcomes of hospital-acquired pressure ulcers and falls. NDNQI helps hospitals benchmark nationally with like units in facilities of the same size and structure (such as academic medical centers or community-based hospitals). Since NDNQI reports are provided at the unit level, a hospital can benchmark with units that are of similar specialty within a defined number of beds. Here's how one organization used NDNQI data to stimulate improvement.

In 2007, based on NDNQI's first quarter results, an intensive care unit (ICU) recognized it had twice the national average of hospital-acquired pressure ulcers. At the same time, Medicare and other payors announced that, beginning the following year, costs for hospital-acquired pressure ulcers would not be covered. This motivated an interdisciplinary team of staff nurses, management, physical therapists, and dieticians to meet and develop an action plan to decrease the number of hospital-acquired pressure ulcers from 40% to 11% within 90 days. The team created a fishbone diagram (Figure 8-1) that showed the areas to be addressed (Morehead, 2008).

Figure 8-1. Pressure Ulcer Fishbone

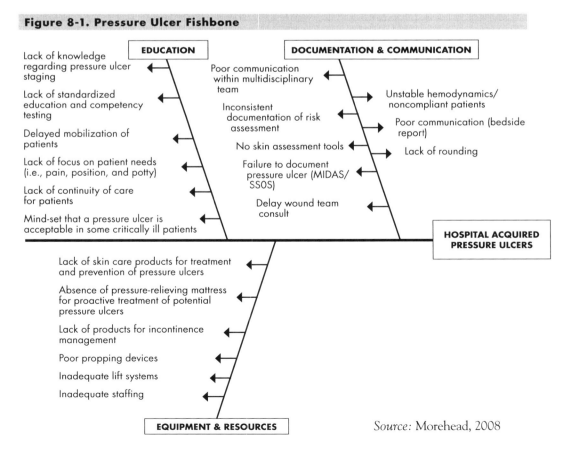

Source: Morehead, 2008

After completing the fishbone diagram, the team developed a Pareto diagram, Figure 8-2, related to the causes of pressure ulcers and skin breakdown.

Figure 8-2. Pareto Diagram: Causes of Hospital-Acquired Pressure Ulcers

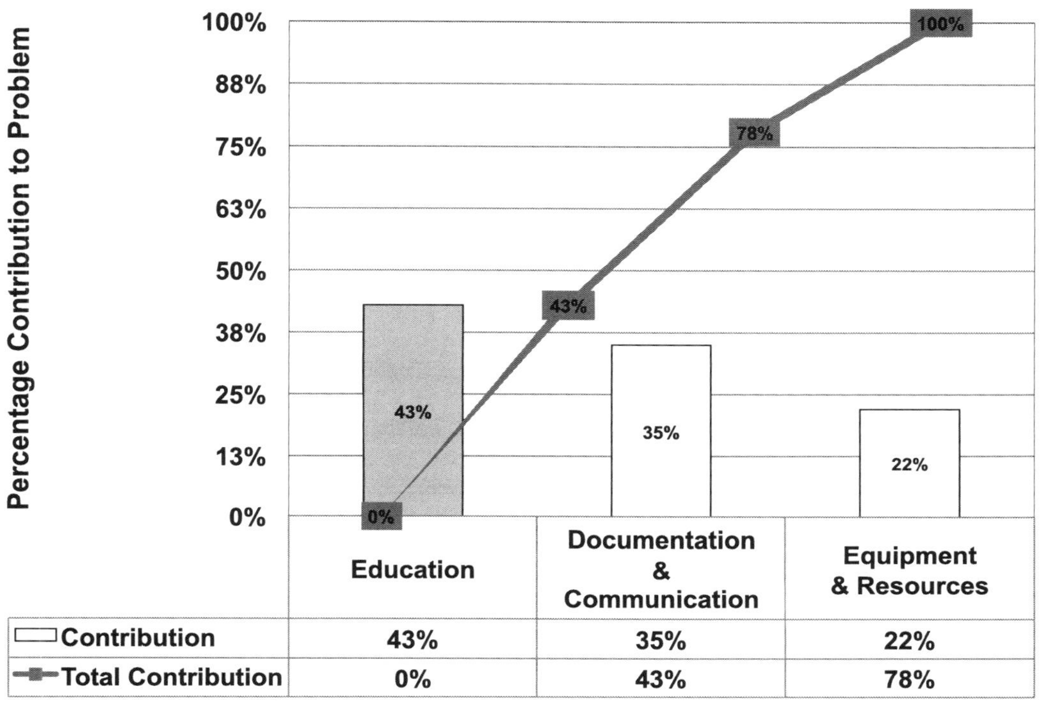

	Education	Documentation & Communication	Equipment & Resources
☐ Contribution	43%	35%	22%
■ Total Contribution	0%	43%	78%

Source: Morehead, 2008

The Pareto diagram helped the team prioritize opportunities to formulate an action plan adapted from the "plan, do, study, act" (PDSA) model. This model PDCA (plan-do-check-act) is an "iterative four-step problem-solving process typically used in business process improvement. It is also known as the Deming cycle, Shewhart cycle, Deming wheel, or plan-do-study-act" model (HCi, 2010) and has been promoted by the Institute for Healthcare Improvement (IHI). After the PDSA action plan was put into practice in the ICU and the desired results were acquired and maintained, the plan was implemented throughout the hospital. The education portion was expanded to eight nursing units. All RNs were required to complete the NDNQI education module for pressure ulcer staging and assessment. A skin and wound assessment tool developed by the ICU staff was incorporated into the critical care flow sheets. The off-going and in-coming nurses were required to assess the patient's skin together at change of shift. The ICU maintained a 0% incidence and prevalence rate of pressure ulcers for 15 months. The initiative created a significant shift in the nurses' mindset that pressure ulcers can be prevented even in the sickest patient populations.

The results were dramatic, as shown in Figure 8-3, resulting in a 0% level of pressure ulcers within one year.

Figure 8-3. Results: Hospital-Acquired Pressure Ulcers

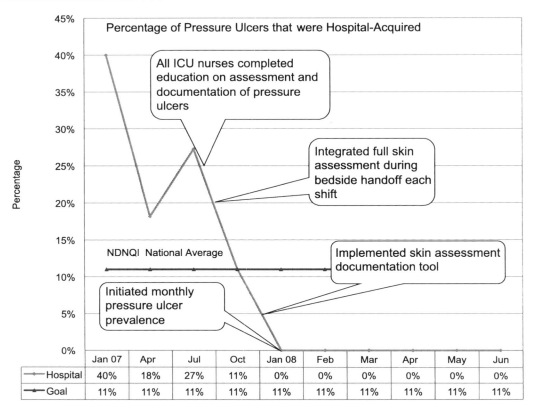

	Jan 07	Apr	Jul	Oct	Jan 08	Feb	Mar	Apr	May	Jun
Hospital	40%	18%	27%	11%	0%	0%	0%	0%	0%	0%
Goal	11%	11%	11%	11%	11%	11%	11%	11%	11%	11%

Source: Morehead, 2008

Comparing their outcomes with peer organizations spurs staff to create a better environment for their patients. Without valid and reliable metrics, improvement efforts often are not productive. The new Magnet Model requires organizations to benchmark and constantly strive to improve structure and processes to yield improved outcomes. Here is another example of how a small community hospital used metrics and benchmarking to improve emergency department (ED) efficiency.

The goal of a small community hospital was to reduce the percentage of patients who left the emergency department (ED) without treatment. Staff took an active role in both redesigning the ED space and changing the triage process to put patients in available rooms sooner. These improvements resulted not only in a significant reduction in patients who left without treatment, but also contributed more than $1 million in additional revenue annually (Figure 8-4).

Figure 8-4. Emergency Department-Left Without Treatment (LWOT) Rate

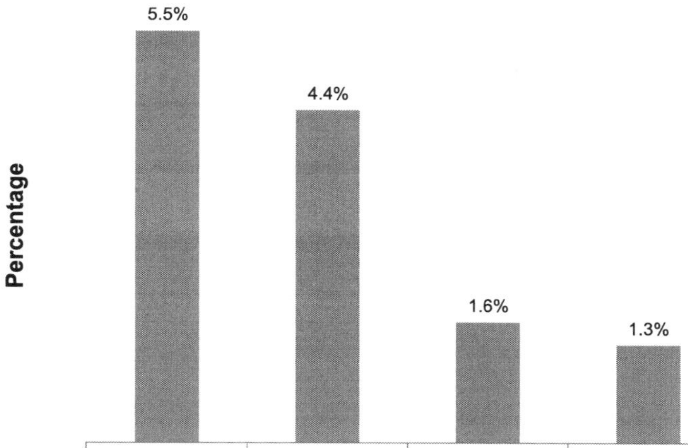

	FY06	FY07	FY08	FY09
▪ LWOT rate	5.5%	4.4%	1.6%	1.3%

Source: Powell, 2008

The redesign also led to momentous improvement in patient satisfaction—all the way from the 9th percentile to the 99th percentile when benchmarked externally to similar-sized hospitals (Figure 8-5).

Figure 8-5. Patient Satisfaction—Percentage Ranking

Patient Satisfaction Ranking

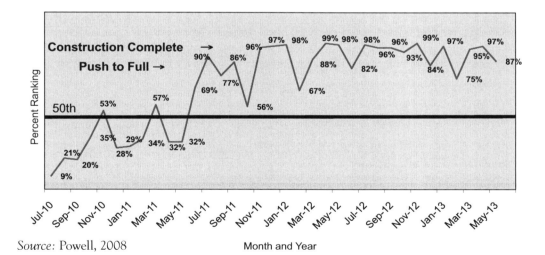

Source: Powell, 2008   Month and Year

The chief nursing officer (CNO) plays a pivotal role in driving evidence-based processes, which result in excellent patient outcomes. The CNO must provide a vision of what ideal practice can be, and use benchmarking to drive improvement. Other responsibilities include freeing up resources for data capture and analysis, development of staff skills in process improvement, and library or list search availability. To improve outcomes for patient, staff, and the community at large, the CNO must be in alignment with other leaders and disciplines and be able to influence change. Direct-care nurses have a responsibility to continuously improve care based on a sense of inquiry. These nurses must have access to databases, know how to use them, and apply evidence-based practices to their patient care. The CNO is the transformational leader who inspires the direct-care nurse to constantly strive to provide the innovative care that patients want and deserve.

SUMMARY

The evolution of the provision of medical and nursing care over the last five decades has a strong link to financial incentives, and systems of care have been organized to take advantage of the flow of finances. This is beginning to change, as the healthcare reform work of this decade will leverage insurance reform as a preliminary first step in transforming the healthcare models by which nurses currently practice. Inherent as a guiding principle in the reform efforts is a link between cost and value. It will no longer be sustainable to pay for any and all care activities; the future payment will be tied to positive patient outcomes and the choices of treatment options will be based on the comparative effectiveness of treatment modalities. For nursing as a discipline, this has far-reaching implications, including the presentation of strong data and research demonstrating the contribution that nursing care provides to patient outcomes. Nursing assessment, interventions, evaluation, and care planning processes are distinctly linked to both prevention of adverse outcomes and promotion of positive healthcare outcomes in every area of health care. As the healthcare reform agenda moves from policy to implementation in practice, the role of the nurse will be more clearly defined as essential to the attainment of positive patient outcomes that will be required.

The new Magnet model places greater emphasis than ever before on measurement and improvement in defined outcomes. This push toward value-based care is congruent with visionaries who stress that mandatory measurement and reporting of patient results, along with higher levels of quality care, are the most important steps in reforming care and lowering costs (Porter & Teisberg, 2006). Transformational leaders are compelled to continually measure and drive improvements. The Magnet framework and focus on outcomes gives all clinicians the capability of practicing at the highest level possible, and ensures that all clinicians are transformational in their work.

REFERENCES

All URLs retrieved September 12, 2010.

American Nurses Credentialing Center. (2008). *Application manual: Magnet Recognition Program.* Silver Spring, MD: Author.

Berwick, D. M. (1989). E. A. Codman and the rhetoric of battle: A commentary. *Milbank Quarterly, 67*(2), 262–267.

Donabedian, A. (1989). The end results of health care: Ernest Codman's contribution to quality assessment and beyond. *Milbank Quarterly, 67*(2), 233–256.

HCi Professional Services. (2010). *PDCA cycle.* Retrieved from http://www.hci.com.au/hcisite3/toolkit/pdcacycl.htm

Institute of Medicine (IOM). (2000). *To err is human: Building a safer health system.* Washington, DC: National Academies Press.

Institute of Medicine (IOM). (2001). *Crossing the quality chasm: A new health system for the 21st century.* Washington, DC: National Academies Press.

Kizlik, Bob. (2010). *Characteristics of a profession.* Retrieved from http://www.adprima.com/profession.htm

Kopf, E. W. (1916). Florence Nightingale as statistician. *Journal of the American Statistical Association, 15,* 388–404.

Morehead, D. (2008). *Reduction in ICU-acquired pressure ulcers.* Storyboard presenation, Baylor Health Care System. Orlando, FL: Institute for Healthcare Improvement.

Neuhauser, D. (1990). Ernest Amory Codman, MD, and end results of medical care. *International Journal of Technology Assessment in Health Care, 6*(2), 307–325.

Nightingale, F. (1863). *Notes on hospitals.* London, England: Longman.

Porter, M. & Teisberg, E. (2006). *Redefining health care: Creating value-based competition on results.* Boston, MA: Harvard Business School Press.

Powell, K. (2008). *Improving care in the emergency department.* Storyboard presentation. Baylor Health Care System. Orlando, FL: Institute for Healthccare Improvement.

Spiegelhalter, D. J. (1999). Surgical audit: Statistical lessons from Nightingale and Codman. *Journal of the Royal Statistical Society, Series A, 162*(1), 45–58.

9

Global Expansion

Karen Drenkard, PhD, RN, NEA-BC, FAAN
Stephanie L. Ferguson, PhD, RN, FAAN
Jeanne Floyd, PhD, RN, CAE

When it comes to global health, there is no "them" ... only "us."
Global Health Council

INTRODUCTION

The nursing shortage is not contained to the United States. There is a similar dearth of qualified nurses in many countries (Buchan & Aiken, 2008; ICN 2005, 2007). Nurses' migration patterns often compound the problem; many countries see their qualified healthcare professionals leave in search of higher wages, better career opportunities, and the excitement of travel. The original Magnet® research (McClure et al., 1983) aimed to identify not what was *wrong* with nursing work environments, but what was *right* with them. It's no wonder, then, that other nations around the world are interested in the Journey to Magnet Excellence™ (Floyd, 2006). To meet this growing level of interest, the American Nurses Credentialing Center (ANCC) is reaching out to healthcare organizations in countries around the world, as they look for ways to decrease RN turnover, lower vacancy rates, and improve the quality of health care.

MAGNET'S GLOBAL EXPANSION

In 1999, responding to increased global credentialing activities, ANCC created Credentialing International. Earlier that year, the International Council of Nurses (ICN) had launched a standard-setting initiative for international distance education; approval of continuing education at the local, national, and international levels; international nurse consultation; accreditation of programs with international components; and certification of nurses and other healthcare professionals as international consultants.

Also in 1999, ANCC began a pilot project with Rochdale Healthcare National Health Service (NHS) Trust in England. The purpose was to gain vital information and establish the foundation for expanding Magnet overseas.

As part of the project, ANCC formed the Magnet Modification Task Force, which included international nurses to review the program and propose global modifications and innovations. The Task Force recommended that Magnet standards and measurement criteria apply to all countries, but that variability be introduced to the interpretive evidence and on-site verification levels. It also recognized that procedures must accommodate application review by equals, i.e., experts in the field who understood and could interpret the context as an expression of peer review. ANCC then convened an international credentialing advisory group to gather information about the global environment, update leadership on international program developments, and promote the international program to the ANCC Board.

In 2001, ANCC collaborated with Linda Aiken and her research team to evaluate efforts to strengthen professional nursing practice in hospitals in Russia and Armenia. Shortly after the fall of the Soviet Union, the U.S. Agency for International Development (USAID) implemented the American International Health Alliance (AIHA) Health Care Partnership Model, which paired Magnet-recognized facilities with hospitals in the country's newly independent states. The partnerships with Magnet-recognized hospitals were meant to develop professional nursing practice in emerging nations. Chief nursing officers at three sites in Russia and two in Armenia selected two of the Forces of Magnetism to explore and implement in their respective environments. Over the next two years, Magnet hospital staff mentored the nurses to assist them to sutccessfully apply the selected Forces of Magnetism. Dr. Aiken's study found that each participating facility had improved patient care quality and the overall care environment. She and her team concluded that the change represented a transformational intervention that served as a catalyst for elevating the workforce and patient care outcomes (Aiken & Poghosyan, 2009).

Meanwhile, ANCC's pilot with Rochdale Healthcare NHS Trust, which earned Magnet designation in 2002, confirmed that the tenets of the Magnet program were culturally transferable. The pilot demonstrated an international applicant's successful use of a hospital advisory committee, and it led to two significant developments: a Magnet glossary to enhance understanding of terms, and the use of advisors to provide the Commission On Magnet (COM) and Magnet appraisers an understanding of the context within which the applicant healthcare organization exists and its nurses practice.

As a result, in 2002 ANCC's International Advisory Council (IAC) was established. This group was composed of nurse leaders from around the world. The IAC would position ANCC as a global leader in providing credentialing programs that directly link professional development and recognition with the practice of quality health care and the development of global alliances to that effect.

In 2000, a Task Force was developed under the leadership of Dr. Margretta Madden Styles. This Task Force was created to assist international aspirant facilities in assessing their Magnet readiness, and provided benchmarks and other support during the Magnet journey. The Magnet Modifcation Task Force was a working unit of the Rochdale Healthcare NHS Trust Pilot Project. It included ANCC's president and representatives from the COM, Magnet hospitals, and the international market. It made the following recommendations to enhance the Magnet program's global applicability:

- Develop consistency and a tiered approach in defining the terminology of assessment—standards, measurement criteria, interpretive evidence, and appraiser scoring guidelines.
- Standardize measurement criteria across healthcare settings and nations—differentiation would appear as needed within interpretive evidence and appraiser scoring guidelines.
- Make accommodations for measurement criteria that are not appropriate for a setting or nation—differences would be noted by parentheses, footnotes, glossaries, and interpretive evidence.
- Develop an instrument to identify gaps in a facility's readiness to achieve Magnet status.

In 2006, ANCC replaced the IAC with the Institute for Credentialing International. Representatives hailed from Australia, Canada, Denmark, Iceland, Ireland, Japan, Korea, New Zealand, the United Kingdom, and the United States. Fadwa Affara, former IAC co-chairperson, and Dr. Cecilia Mulvey, ANCC's immediate past president, co-chaired the Institute's Governing Council. After three years of significant contribution to ANCC, the Governing Council completed its term in 2009 and global representation was mainstreamed throughout ANCC.

PLANNING ASSUMPTIONS

In 2009, a decision was made by the ANCC Board of Directors to pro-actively determine the plan for international growth and expansion of the Magnet Recognition Program. Before developing a business plan for Magnet expansion into global markets, ANCC addressed several key assumptions:

- Service and quality must remain the same.
- Appraiser competency, quality, consistency, and service must remain the same.
- Hospitals around the globe must use the new outcome-focused, evidence-based Magnet model.
- If necessary, services and tools to assist with the Magnet application should be redesigned to address cultural differences in a country or region.
- On-line submission of the Demographic Information Form (DIF) and Magnet application must remain the same.
- The COM's decision-making process regarding Magnet status must remain the same.
- Governance remains under ANCC control.
- It is anticipated that international growth trajectories of the Magnet program will mirror domestic growth rates.

In addition, ANCC assumed the following considerations for decisions about the choice of model:

- Size of country and number and size of hospitals or other health agencies, (e.g., ambulatory care, nursing homes);

- Capacity to develop professional nursing within cultural boundaries, including consideration of regulations, licensure, education, and continuing education;
- Financial sustainability of country;
- Quality of healthcare organizations within the country;
- Capability to collect data, including definitions, and technology infrastructure;
- Safety of the region; and
- Ethical and social justice.

RATIONALE: BENEFITS TO GLOBAL SOCIETIES

Magnet as a program has grown because as a set of standards it serves as a roadmap to achieving nurse retention and satisfaction, excellence in the patient experience, and positive clinical outcomes for quality and safety. These outcomes are applicable to the global community. As Magnet continues to thrive as the only international recognition for nursing excellence in healthcare organizations, the Magnet program is realizing its vision. Both the domestic and international nursing literature cite Magnet status as a solution to the RN shortage and a means to ensure that the safety and quality agenda is achieved. Thus, knowledge of its purpose and characteristics has increased worldwide (Lundmark, 2008). Even with the economic downturn, healthcare organizations recognize that this is the time to invest in quality and patient safety. In fact, in times of turbulence, great opportunities exist to build a foundation for global growth of the Magnet program. As it can take healthcare organizations from two to five years to complete the Magnet journey, the time is right to establish the building blocks for international applicants. Magnet can benefit the global society as it moves toward positive patient outcomes and healthy nations.

Organizations that can demonstrate excellence in quality and patient safety and satisfaction will thrive in a downturn. According to Rhodes and Stelter (2009), "inaction is the riskiest response to the uncertainties of an economic crisis" (p. 51). The same is true for Magnet. An analysis of all countries in the world narrows the focus to a select few that would meet the criteria for the Magnet Recognition Program in their markets.

There are currently (2010) four international Magnet hospitals:
- Princess Alexandra Hospital Health Service District in Australia
- Sir Charles Gairdner Hospital in Australia
- American University of Beirut Medical Center in Lebanon
- Singapore General Hospital in Singapore

In addition, Belgium, Finland, Germany, Canada, Japan, Jordan, Saudi Arabia, South Korea, The Netherlands, and the United Kingdom have expressed interest in Magnet. In a 2009 fact-finding mission with key officials from the ICN, World Health Organization (WHO), International Hospital Federation, European Union, and Health Attaché of the United States Mission to the United Nations, all agreed that Magnet is strategically poised to make a difference for nations that are striving for excellence in nursing, healthcare services, and patient safety. In July 2009, the Board of Directors of ANCC voted to approve a business plan to target three regions of the world for growth: European Union, Eastern Mediterranean, and Western Pacific.

The most recent World Health Organization (WHO) resolution, WHA 59.27, gives the WHO the mandate to strengthen the capacity of the nursing and midwifery workforce through the provision of support to member states on:

- "Establishing comprehensive programs for the development of human resources for health, which support recruitment and retention of sufficient numbers in the nursing and midwifery workforce;
- Involvement of nurses and midwives in the development of their health systems;
- Country-level implementation of the WHO's strategic directions for nursing and midwifery;
- Regular review of the legislation and regulatory processes;
- Collection and use of nursing and midwifery core data; and
- Development and implementation of ethical recruitment of national and international nursing and midwifery workforce" (WHO, 2008).

These recommendations (WHO, 2006a, pp. 38–40) are aligned with Magnet standards and underscore how such standards can serve as a mechanism to improve healthcare quality in the global market.

The Strategic Directions for Nursing and Midwifery Services, developed by the WHO and its partners (2002–2008), provide a framework for collaborative action to enhance nursing and midwifery services that contribute to achieving both national health goals and the health-related Millennium Development Goals (MDGs) of the United Nations system. The main strategic areas are:

- Health planning, advocacy, and political commitment
- Management of health personnel for nursing and midwifery services
- Practice and health systems improvement
- Education of health personnel for nursing and midwifery services
- Stewardship and governance

The Journey to Magnet Excellence™ can strengthen all of these strategic areas and make significant headway in the enhancement of nursing and midwifery services.

The Agency for Healthcare Research and Quality included Magnet outcomes in its most recent compendium for patient quality and safety (Lundmark, 2008). This affirms the contribution of the Magnet Recognition Program toward improving patient care. With maturity well established in the United States, Magnet has a responsibility to contribute to the worldwide improvement of patient outcomes.

Global mandates to relieve shortages and imbalances in the nursing workforce, improve nurses' professional development, move health environments toward positive practice and incentives, move the nursing profession toward evidence-based practice, and require strong nursing standards and ethics have increased interest in the Magnet Recognition Program (Burdett Project, ICN, 2005). The Magnet Recognition Program is the roadmap for organizations that are striving to meet these mandates. Magnet will contribute significantly to the achievement and sustainability of nursing excellence and delivery of patient care around the world.

As validated by growing amounts of research, the Magnet Recognition Program adds credibility and evidence to the global quest for patient safety and quality health care (Lundmark, 2008). Magnet is unique in that it focuses on nurses and nursing services as the touchstone for quality and safety in healthcare systems. As the largest group of health professionals, nurses are the backbone of healthcare delivery systems in most nations in the world (WHO, 2006a). Yet, as a result of shortages and migration of nursing staff, hospitals around the globe are struggling to maintain their standards and attract and retain nurses (WHO, 2006). Magnet recognition provides a professional development framework to improve the recruitment and retention of nurses and the creation and sustainability of positive practice environments. The program's platform and components establish criteria such as:

- Shared governance structures
- Strong nursing ethics
- Principles of Transformational Leadership
- Autonomy and respect in nursing practice, regulation, and education (including nursing registration and credentialing at the BSN, MSN, and advanced-practice levels)
- Ongoing nursing research and practice that is evidence- and outcome-based

In the recent publication, *Guidelines: Incentives for Health Professionals*, the authors note (Global Health Alliance, 2008) that there are both financial and non-financial incentives for the improved retention of healthcare professionals, especially nurses. Magnet-recognized hospitals create an opportunity for nurses to actively pursue all of these elements. The financial indicators include traditional incentives to improve working conditions for nurses, such as wages, benefits (conditions), and performance-linked payments. However, both the Magnet journey and Magnet recognition can help hospitals and organizations worldwide to not only survive, but also thrive, while achieving a balance of incentives—including non-financial ones—for nurse development and growth. These include career and professional development, workload management, flexible working arrangements, positive working environments, and access to benefits and supports such as continuing nursing education opportunities. In Magnet-recognized facilities, nurse retention improves as the investment includes not just financial rewards, but also career development and growth. Increasingly, research is demonstrating that the result of improved nurse retention is improved patient outcomes.

Health systems that offer nurses these incentives become "magnets" for RNs and beacons for quality patient care. Successful and satisfied nurses create a synergy toward positive change, which impacts the entire healthcare system. Nurses set the course for day-to-day excellence.

ANCC recently surveyed its Magnet appraisers to determine their international experience, foreign language capabilities, recommendations for cultural transferability of the Sources of Evidence and FOM, and the data collection, consultation, and education services needed for successful global expansion. The first group of appraisers had conducted site visits and surveyed facilities in Australia, New Zealand, and Lebanon. All noted that the FOM were relevant in their international experiences. What surprised the appraisers most during their visits was how similar the countries' health systems and nursing issues were to those in the United States. In some instances, the appraisers were impressed by how advanced nursing care delivery was in these nations. Some of the noted differences included a lack of evolution and integration of ethics, a diminished concept of advanced practice nursing, a decreased level of patient safety overall, and a lack of benchmarking against relevant databases.

Challenges experienced on the international site visits included:
- The need to translate and interpret English.
- Understanding each country's healthcare system in general.

- Assessing the Sources of Evidence within the context of each country's healthcare system—for example, because advanced practice nursing is in a very early stage of development in Australia, its relationship to the Sources of Evidence is quite different from that in the United States.

Sources of Evidence that described different processes included standards related to nursing peer review, governance and operational structures, and the role of credentialing and privileging processes in advanced practice nursing. Interestingly, the process descriptions addressed all of the required Sources of Evidence for Magnet designation.

Other recommendations from the international appraisers that are in the process of being implemented include:

- Conference calls and planning meetings with international advisors prior to the site visit are helpful to learn more about local demographics, health care, and nursing care, and to place the Sources of Evidence in context.
- Appraisers need to have a broad perspective on how each nation's health system works, especially regarding care of indigenous populations.
- Even in English-speaking countries, language interpretation can be challenging due to dialects. Continued clarification of conversations is critical.
- As noted above, it is important to focus on the Sources of Evidence in the context of each nation and its particular evidence and data.
- The Organizational Overview (OO) or Demographic Information Form (DIF) should add a section for the international applicant to describe the country's healthcare system and how the hospital fits in that system (government-owned, government-run, publicly or privately funded, etc.).
- In many nations, there are multiple government reports that appraisers should review prior to the site visit. These reports guide the organization and nursing departments' strategic and quality plans.
- Sources of Evidence that need global interpretation include nursing governance, nursing peer review, and advanced practice nurse credentialing and privileging.
- A separate appendix should be added to the Magnet manual to address issues related to international applications.
- The Magnet manual glossary should be expanded to include global definitions on nursing governance, peer review, advanced practice nurse credentialing and privileging, and basic definitions related to global healthcare systems.
- Further preparation is needed for appraisers working in global markets and performing international site visits. Such preparation should include the current practice of conference calls with Magnet staff and international advisers, as well as planning sessions with the Magnet team before actual site visits.

In addition to the international appraisers' survey, ANCC surveyed its current pool of domestic Magnet appraisers. This survey focused on their interest in international work; language capacity; recommendations for cultural transferability of Sources of Evidence, the OO, and the DIF; and recommendations for appraiser capacity building in the context of Magnet's global expansion.

THE WAY FORWARD

Magnet staff assessed the survey results and added a new international appendix to the Magnet manual. Survey findings will continue to impact development of international application material and processes, including appraiser visits and appraisers' educational needs.

As part of the current international application process, the Magnet Program Office conducts an in-depth conference call with each organization to validate eligibility. In addition, a dedicated team of international analysts and specialists assists in all phases of the application process to ensure that organizations understand and accurately interpret the intent of the Sources of Evidence.

International organizations must collect data reflecting nurse and patient satisfaction and other nurse-sensitive clinical outcomes at the unit level. The data must be compared against national benchmarks. In some countries, this is difficult to achieve because there are no comparative benchmarks. The Magnet Program Office works with applicants to determine the best source of comparative data and to make recommendations of viable options. Documents will continue to be submitted in English. All site visit requirements are the same for international applicants. However, it is important that staff have an opportunity to speak in their own language. While highly qualified international appraisers are assigned for document and site visit review, they may not be fluent in the language the organization uses. Mutually agreed-upon interpreters and translators may be used during the site visit. The translators and interpreters must work for ANCC through a service agreement, as all Magnet materials and products are copyrighted and trademarked. All costs associated with this service are the applicant's responsibility.

ANCC has added three international members to the COM, which is ultimately responsible for bestowing the Magnet credential. The new members are Franz Wagner, CEO, German Nurses Association and former first vice president, International Council of Nurses; Veronica Casey, former chief nurse, Princess Alexandra Hospital in Australia; and Gladys Mouro, chief nurse, American University of Beirut Medical Center in Lebanon.

The Magnet Recognition Program has the flexibility necessary to meet the needs of global health institutions and celebrate those that provide a positive work environment, excellent nursing services, and quality health care for all. Achieving Magnet recognition is neither a project nor an award, but rather a credential that recognizes excellence in nursing care. A Magnet culture is a way of life for nursing practice and the actual provision of nursing care in healthcare organizations that make a commitment to excellence. "To be effective, the Chief Nurse Executive has to be the role model for living the tenets in Magnet's core components and principles" (Drenkard, 2005, p. 221). Further, Drenkard notes that the work of Magnet is the work of all the nurses within an organization, and a culture of "magnetism" has a spirit of shared governance and leadership, peer accountability, and a continuous desire to improve the work environment (p. 222).

Celebrating milestones is a core tenet of Magnet; ANCC is celebrating more than a decade in which its mission to promote excellence in nursing and health care through credentialing programs and related services has caught on around the world (Floyd, 2006). This has the potential to stabilize the global nursing workforce with improved RN recruitment and retention, and to boost the professional image of nursing worldwide. What does the future hold? Tremendous potential to learn from other cultures and to transfer knowledge across cultures.

REFERENCES

All URLs retrieved September 12, 2010.

Aiken, L. H., & Poghosyan, L. (2009). Evaluation of "Magnet journey to nursing excellence program" in Russia and Armenia. *Journal of Nursing Scholarship, 41*(2), 166–174.

Buchan, J., & Aiken, L. H. (2008). Solving nursing shortages: A common priority. *Journal of Clinical Nursing, 17*(24), 3262–3268.

Drenkard, K. (2005). Sustaining Magnet: Keeping the forces alive. *Nursing Administration Quarterly, 29*(3), 214–222.

Floyd, J. (2006). Innovations in health care delivery: Responses to global nurse migration—A practice example. *Policy, Politics, & Nursing Practice, 7*(3), 44S–48S.

Global Health Workforce Alliance. (2008). *Guidelines: Incentives for health professionals.* Global Positive Practice Environment Campaign. Retrieved from http://www.ihf-fih.org/pdf/Incentives_Guidelines%20EN.PDF

International Council of Nurses (ICN). (2007). *Positive practice environments: Quality workplaces = quality patient care.* Retrieved from http://www.icn.ch/publications/2007-positive-practice-environments-quality-workplaces-quality-patient-care/

Lundmark, V. (2008). Magnet environments for professional nursing practice. In R. G. Hughes (Ed.), *Patient safety and quality: An evidence-based handbook for nurses.* Rockville, MD: Agency for Healthcare Research and Quality.

McClure, M., Poulin, M., Sovie, M., & Wandelt, M. (1983). *Magnet hospitals: Attraction and retention of professional nurses.* Kansas City, MO: American Nurses Association.

Rhodes, D., & Stelter, D. (2009). Seize advantage in a downturn. *Harvard Business Review, 87*(2), 50–58.

World Health Organization (WHO). (2006a). *The world health report 2006: Working together for health.* Retrieved from http://www.who.int/whr/2006/en/index.html

World Health Organization (WHO). (2006b). *The global shortage of health workers and its impact.* Fact Sheet No. 302. Retrieved from http://www.who.int/workforcealliance/knowledge/resources/workforcecrisis_factsheet/en/index.html

World Health Organization (WHO). (2007). *Global patient safety challenge.* World Alliance for Patient Safety Programme. Retrieved from http://www.who.int/patientsafety/challenge/en/

World Health Organization (WHO). (2008). *Nursing and midwifery at WHO.* Retrieved from http://www.who.int/hrh/nursing_midwifery/en/

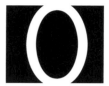

Magnet Practice Environments and Outcomes

Vicki A. Lundmark, PhD
Joanne V. Hickey, PhD, APRN-BC, ACNP, FAAN, FCCM

Knowledge itself is power.
Sir Francis Bacon

INTRODUCTION

This chapter reviews recent research connecting Magnet® environments for professional nursing practice to workforce, organizational, or patient outcomes, and discusses the need for further research in this area. The chapter includes an update to the literature (Lundmark, 2008), which was conducted four years ago and is reproduced in this volume as an appendix (starting on p. 139). Compared to findings from the previous review, the present review shows both that the pace of research on these topics has accelerated and that the research methodologies have improved.

The systematic review contained in this chapter's appendix (titled Magnet Environments for Professional Nursing Practice) was conducted in 2006 and encompassed 31 research articles that reported results from primary or secondary data analysis and included nurse or patient outcome variables. The reviewed articles were published from 1987 to 2006. During that time, the evidence linking Magnet environments to the quality of patient care appeared to be promising but limited. While findings tended to demonstrate consistent relationships between Magnet characteristics and favorable nurse or patient outcomes, most of the research to date had employed subjective methods. Nearly all of the 31 studies reviewed had relied solely on cross-sectional survey data from staff nurses. Thus, the most commonly used measure to represent patient outcomes was nurse perception of the quality of care. The review concluded that researchers would need to raise the level of theoretical and methodological sophistication to fully understand the mechanisms that connect nursing environments to patient outcomes.

RECENT RESEARCH FINDINGS

Articles in this review were primarily identified by electronic searches of medical and social science reference databases[1] and occasionally by personal referral through colleagues. To locate potential review articles, two sets of search terms were used. Various combinations of the words *magnet* or *magnetism* and *nurse* or *nursing* constituted the first set of search terms. The second set of search terms was employed to locate studies that had used one of the practice environment measurement instruments associated with Magnet characteristics, which are itemized in Table 10-1.

Table 10-1. Instruments Measuring Magnet Environment Characteristics

Article	Instrument	Subscales
Aiken & Patrician, 2000	Nursing Work Index-Revised (NWI-R) (57 items)	3 subscales and 1 alternate subscale: • Nurse autonomy (5 items) • Control over nursing practice setting (7 items) • Nurse relations with physicians (3 items) • Organizational support (10 of the items above)
Lake, 2002	Practice Environment Scale – Nursing Work Index (PES-NWI) (31 items)	5 subscales: • Nurse participation in hospital affairs (9 items) • Nursing foundations for quality of care (10 items) • Nurse manager ability, leadership, and support of nurses (5 items) • Staffing and resource adequacy (4 items) • Collegial nurse–physician relations (3 items)
Choi et al., 2004	Perceived Nursing Work Environment (PNWE) (42 items)	7 subscales: • Professional practice (13 items) • Staffing and resource adequacy (5 items) • Nurse management (5 items) • Nursing process (6 items) • Nurse–physician collaboration (4 items) • Nurse competence (6 items) • Positive scheduling climate (3 items)

The appendix describes, in some detail, the development of the *Nursing Work Index-Revised (NWI-R)* and its relationship to Magnet characteristics. Survey items constituting the original Nursing Work Index were conceived from the literature on job satisfaction, work values, and the first study of Magnet hospitals published in the early 1980s (Kramer & Hafner, 1989; Lake, 2007; McClure et al., 1983). The NWI-R was adapted from the NWI to measure organizational features and to delineate four subscales (Aiken, 2002; Aiken & Patrician, 2000).

Subsequently, both the *Practice Environment Scale–Nursing Work Index (PES-NWI)* and the *Perceived Nursing Work Environment (PNWE)* instruments were created using the same pool of survey items as the NWI with each one classified through factor analysis into different sets of subscales (Choi et al., 2004; Lake, 2002). In 2004, the National Quality Forum endorsed the PES-NWI as a Nursing Care Performance Measure (National Quality Forum, 2004). As the present review attests, it has become widely disseminated in the research literature (Lake, 2007).

Studies were retained for review if they (a) reported results from primary or secondary data analysis; (b) included variables to represent Magnet environment characteristics or Magnet recognition status; (c) included at least one nurse, workforce, organizational, or patient outcome as an associated or dependent variable; and (d) represented hospital practice settings. Studies investigating the effects of Magnet characteristics in non-hospital settings were excluded as there are reasons to believe that organizational characteristics relate differently to quality of care across diverse healthcare settings (Hearld et al., 2008).

These criteria identified a total of 27 studies. They are listed in Table 10-2 along with a brief description of their size or scope. One article was released as an e-publication ahead of print early in 2010 (Chen & Johantgen, 2010). Otherwise, the publication dates range from 2006 to 2009. The third column in Table 10-2 describes the data sources for each study's outcome measures. Seven studies included outcome variables from objective sources such as discharge data or incident reports, and two studies based outcomes on patient reports.

To highlight the range of Magnet environment and outcome relationships that researchers have investigated, the next three tables itemize the outcome measures of the studies listed in Table 10-2. The tables are organized according to data source—those with outcomes based on nurse surveys (Table 10-3), patient reports (Table 10-4), and organizational data (Table 10-5). However, it should be noted that the majority of studies reviewed examined the influence of Magnet factors in combination with additional independent variables of major or primary interest. Compared to the majority of studies reviewed in this chapter's appendix, which tended to rely on bivariate comparisons and small numbers of variables, this is one of the ways the research has progressed.

STUDIES WITH OUTCOMES BASED ON NURSE SURVEYS

Many studies have focused on nurse-reported outcome measures such as job satisfaction, intent to leave, and nurse perceptions of care quality or safety. Table 10-3, which is grouped by type of Magnet measure, lists the associated or dependent variables for studies with outcomes based on nurse surveys. Findings from the studies are described below.

Job Satisfaction

Magnet to Non-Magnet Comparisons
Table 10-3 lists five studies that compared job satisfaction between nurses in Magnet-recognized organizations and nurses in non-Magnet organizations. All but one found significant associations. Four studies (Lacey et al., 2007; Schmalenberg et al., 2008;

Table 10-2. Studies Reviewed for This Chapter

Article	Sample	Outcomes Data Sources
Aiken et al., 2008	10,184 nurses, 232,342 patients, 168 Pennsylvania hospitals	Nurse survey, discharge data
Armstrong et al., 2008	153 nurses, Ontario	Nurse survey
Chen & Johantgen, 2010	3,182 RNs, 31 acute care hospitals, Germany & Belgium	Nurse survey
Clarke, 2007	11,512 RNs, 188 Pennsylvania hospitals	Nurse survey
Dunton et al., 2007	1,610 units, >1,100 U.S. hospitals	Unit reports
Friese et al., 2008	<10,184 RNs, 24,618 patients, 164 Pennsylvania hospitals	Discharge data
Hughes et al., 2009	3,689 RNs, 286 medical-surgical units, 146 acute care hospitals	Nurse survey
Kim et al., 2009	192 RNs, 3 New York hospitals	Nurse survey
Kovner et al., 2009	1,406 newly licensed RNs, 34 states & DC	Nurse survey
Kutney-Lee et al., 2009	20,984 RNs, ≈100,000 patients, 430 hospitals (CA, PA, NJ, FL)	Patient survey
Lacey et al., 2007	3,337 nurses, 292 units, 15 institutions, 11 states	Nurse survey
Laschinger, 2008	234 nurses, Ontario hospitals	Nurse survey
Manojlovich, 2005	284 hospital-based nurses, Michigan hospitals	Nurse survey
Manojlovich et al., 2009	462 ICU nurses, 25 units, 8 Michigan hospitals	Administrative data
Manojlovich & DeCicco, 2007	445 ICU nurses, 25 units, 8 Michigan hospitals	Nurse survey
Manojlovich & Laschinger, 2007	276 nurses, Michigan	Nurse survey
Schmalenberg & Kramer, 2008	10,514 staff nurses, 34 U.S. hospitals	Nurse survey
Seago, 2008	314 nurses, 470 patients, 60 units, 21 California hospitals	Patient interview
Siu et al., 2008	678 RNs, 148 units, 9 Ontario hospitals	Nurse survey
Stone & Gershon, 2006	837 nurses, 39 ICUs, 23 U.S. hospitals	Incident reports
Stone, Mooney-Kane, Larson, Pastor, et al., 2007 [Med Care]	1,095 nurses, 15,846 patients, 51 adult ICUs, 31 U.S. hospitals	Infection data, Medicare data
Stone, Mooney-Kane, Larson, Horan, et al., 2007 [HSR]	837 nurses, 39 ICUs, 23 hospitals, 20 U.S. metropolitan areas	Nurse survey
Tourangeau et al., 2006	3,886 RNs & RPNs, 46,933 patients, 75 hospitals, Ontario	Discharge data
Ulrich, Buerhaus, et al., 2007	735 newly licensed RNs in U.S.	Nurse survey
Ulrich, Woods, et al., 2007	3,332 critical care nurses	Nurse survey
Wade et al., 2008	731 RNs in a large mid-Atlantic health system	Nurse survey

Ulrich, Buerhaus et al., 2007; Ulrich, Woods et al., 2007) found that nurses in Magnet organizations were significantly more satisfied than nurses in non-Magnet organizations. The fifth study (Kovner et al., 2009), found no association between Magnet status and satisfaction.

Three of these studies included an additional comparison group: nurses from "Magnet-aspiring" organizations. Two of the studies (Lacey et al., 2007; Ulrich, Woods et al., 2007) found that nurses in Magnet-aspiring organizations had significantly higher satisfaction rates than nurses in non-Magnet organizations. The third study (Ulrich, Buerhaus et al., 2007) found that nurses in Magnet-aspiring organizations and nurses in non-Magnet organizations were about equally satisfied.

PES-NWI Comparisons

Four job satisfaction studies listed in Table 10-3 measured Magnet characteristics through the PES-NWI and reported findings at the subscale level. Positive associations between the environment components and job satisfaction were found in nearly every case. Two studies (Laschinger, 2008; Manojlovich & Laschinger, 2007) found that all five PES-NWI subscale components related favorably to each other and to work satisfaction in path analysis modeling. Another study (Wade et al., 2008) found that all PES-NWI subscale components related significantly to job enjoyment except for one: nurse participation in hospital affairs. The last of the four studies (Kovner et al., 2009), which included only one of the PES-NWI subscales among its measures, found a significant association between nurse–physician relations and job satisfaction.

Two of the job satisfaction studies in this group employed some form of a composite PES-NWI score as a single variable. Both found significant positive relationships between practice environment and satisfaction. In one (Aiken et al., 2008), only three PES-NWI subscale components were used to reduce overlap with additional independent variables, and results showed that more positive environments were linked to lower burnout. In the other (Manojlovich, 2005), all five PES-NWI subscale components were used to form the composite measure.

The last study listed in Table 10-3 (Chen & Johantgen, 2010) used 23 survey items from the European Nurses Early Exit (NEXT) Study to represent six Magnet characteristics. This analysis found that all six Magnet factors significantly predicted job satisfaction at the nurse level, and that all but two characteristics (quality of nursing leadership and personnel policies) significantly predicted job satisfaction at the hospital level. At the nurse level, personnel policies had the strongest effect in predicting job satisfaction; at the hospital level, management style was strongest.

Intent to Leave

Magnet to Non-Magnet Comparisons

Two studies listed in Table 10-3 examined differences in intent to leave between nurses in Magnet organizations and nurses in non-Magnet organizations. One found that nurses in non-Magnet organizations were significantly more likely to report plans to leave (Ulrich, Buerhaus et al., 2007), while the other found no relationship between working in a Magnet organization and either intent to stay or organizational commitment (Kovner et al., 2009).

Table 10-3. Studies With Outcomes Based on Nurse Survey: Magnet and Outcome Measures

Article	Magnet Measure(s)	Associated or Dependent Variable(s)	
		Satisfaction and Intent to Leave	*Quality of care and Safety*
Hughes et al., 2009	Magnet recognition		Safety climate
Lacey et al., 2007	Magnet recognition	Workload satisfaction	
Schmalenberg et al., 2008	Magnet recognition	Job satisfaction	Overall quality of care
Ulrich, Buerhaus, et al., 2007	Magnet recognition	Satisfaction with present job Plans to leave	
Ulrich, Woods, et al., 2007	Magnet recognition	Satisfaction with current job	Quality of care
Kovner et al., 2009	Magnet recognition PES/NWI – 1 scale	Job satisfaction Organizational commitment Intent to stay	
Armstrong et al., 2008	PES/NWI – 5 scales composite		Safety climate
Aiken et al., 2008	PES/NWI – 3 scales composite	Burnout Job satisfaction Intent to leave	Quality of Care
Clarke, 2007	PES/NWI – 5 scales and aggregated		Sharps injuries
Kim et al., 2009	PES/NWI – 5 scales		Quality of geriatric care
Laschinger, 2008	PES/NWI – 5 scales	Work satisfaction	Quality of care
Manojlovich, 2005	PES/NWI – 4 scales	Job satisfaction	
Manojlovich & DeCicco, 2007	PES/NWI – 5 scales composite		Frequency of • medication errors • catheter-associated sepsis • ventilator-associated pneumonia
Manojlovich & Laschinger, 2007	PES/NWI – 5 scales	Work satisfaction	
Siu et al., 2008	PES/NWI – 5 scales composite		Unit effectiveness
Stone, Larson, et al., 2006	PNWE – 7 scales	Intent to leave	
Stone, Mooney-Kane, Larson, Pastor, et al., 2007	PNWE – 7 scales and composite	Intent to leave	

Table 10-3. Studies With Outcomes Based on Nurse Survey: Magnet and Outcome Measures (cont.)

Article	Magnet Measure(s)	Associated or Dependent Variable(s)	
		Satisfaction and Intent to Leave	*Quality of care and Safety*
Wade et al., 2008	PES/NWI – 5 scales	Job enjoyment	
Chen & Johantgen, 2010	Six Magnet forces: •Leadership •Management style •Personnel policies •Autonomy •Interdisciplinary relations •Professional development	Job satisfaction	

PES-NWI Comparisons

Three additional studies listed in Table 10-3 investigated relationships between intent to leave and measures formed from the PES-NWI or PNWE scales. The two studies that used composite measures (Aiken et al., 2008; Stone, Mooney-Kane, Larson, Pastor et al., 2007) found that more favorable practice environment levels were associated with less likelihood of reporting intentions to leave. The study that used individual subscales measures (Stone, Larson et al., 2006) found that only two of the seven PNWE subscales—professional practice and nurse competence—had an independent effect on intent to leave due to working conditions.

Quality of Care

Magnet to Non-Magnet Comparisons

Both of the studies in this category (Schmalenberg, 2008; Ulrich, Woods et al., 2007) found nurses in Magnet organizations reporting significantly higher perceptions of quality of care than nurses in non-Magnet organizations. In the study (Ulrich, Woods et al., 2007) that also included a third comparison group, quality of care was similarly rated significantly higher among nurses in Magnet-aspiring organizations than among those in non-Magnet organizations.

PES-NWI Comparisons

Of the four studies in this group, three demonstrated positive associations between practice environment factors and quality of care. Results from the fourth study were mixed. Using composite PES-NWI measures, one study (Aiken et al., 2008) linked more positive practice environments to higher nurse-perceived quality of care, and another (Siu et al., 2008) linked them to unit effectiveness. The measure for unit effectiveness is similar to quality-of-care concepts in that it is composed of survey items representing perceptions of technical quality of care provided in the unit, judgment of the unit's ability to meet family member needs, and nursing turnover in the unit (Shortell et al., 1991). Using individual PES-NWI subscale measures, the third study (Laschinger, 2008) likewise found more positive professional environment factors linked to higher nurse evaluations of the care provided.

The study of PES-NWI factors and geriatric care quality (Kim et al., 2009) produced some counterintuitive results. It found that only nurse participation in hospital affairs was positively and significantly associated with the quality of geriatric care. Two other PES-NWI factors—nursing foundations for quality of care and staffing and resource adequacy—were negatively linked to care quality. No associations with care quality were found for the two PES-NWI factors related to nurse managers and nurse–physician relations.

Safety

Magnet to Non-Magnet Comparisons

The one study in this category (Hughes et al., 2009) yielded mixed results. Using a safety climate[2] measure composed of seven subscales, it found that nurses in Magnet organizations were more likely to openly communicate about errors and to participate in error-related problem solving. However, no differences were found between nurses in Magnet organizations and nurses in non-Magnet organizations on the remaining five subscales: safety compliance, safety-related employee feedback, managerial commitment to safety, workgroup commitment to safety, and willingness to reveal errors.

PES-NWI Comparisons

Results from the three studies in this group are likewise mixed. One (Manojlovich & DeCicco, 2007) found that Magnet characteristics did not predict any of the three nurse-reported adverse events measured. However, the other two found favorable associations between Magnet characteristics and safety-related outcomes. The first study (Armstrong et al., 2008) found all five PES-NWI subscales as well as a total PES-NWI score to be significantly related to safety climate measured as a set of seven survey items. The second study (Clarke, 2007) found that "nurses in the 25 hospitals that were in the top quartile on all or all but one of the five [PES-NWI] work environment scales were 34% less likely to experience an injury" (p. 306).

STUDIES WITH OUTCOMES BASED ON PATIENT REPORTS

Studies with outcome measures based on patient reports appear to be relatively rare.

Patient Satisfaction

PES-NWI Comparisons

Table 10-4 identifies two studies that investigated the association of practice environment factors to patient satisfaction using either PES-NWI or NWI-R scales to measure Magnet characteristics. One (Kutney-Lee et al., 2009) found significant and positive associations between a composite PES-NWI score and all 10 of the HCAHPS (Hospital Consumer Assessment of Healthcare Providers and Systems) patient satisfaction survey questions. In this case, the composite score represented three PES-NWI subscales. Two of those subscales—nurse participation in hospital affairs and staffing and resource adequacy—were excluded because they were highly correlated with other staffing measures used in the study.

The second study in this group (Seago, 2008) uncovered more insignificant or counterintuitive findings than positive ones. None of the four NWI-R subscale factors demonstrated an association to patient satisfaction with pain management or to patient satisfaction with physical care except for nurse relations with physicians, which was positively linked to satisfaction with physical care. The relationships found between NWI-R factors and patient satisfaction with teaching were mixed: control over nursing practice was not associated, organizational support was positively associated, and both autonomy and nurse relations with physicians were negatively associated to satisfaction with teaching.

Table 10-4. Studies With Outcomes Based on Patient Reports: Magnet and Outcome Measures

Article	Magnet Measure(s)	Associated or Dependent Variable(s)
Kutney-Lee et al., 2009	PES/NWI – 3 scales composite	Patient survey: 10 items from HCAHPS (Hospital Consumer Assessment of Healthcare Providers and Systems) survey. For example: • Nurses always communicate well • Staff gave discharge information • Always received help as soon as wanted • Would recommend the hospital
Seago, 2008	NWI-R – 4 scales	Patient interview: • Patient satisfaction with teaching • Patient satisfaction with pain management • Patient satisfaction with physical care

STUDIES WITH OUTCOMES BASED ON ORGANIZATIONAL DATA

The next two tables describe the seven studies that included outcomes based on objective sources. Table 10-5 names the outcome indicators for each study; Table 10-6 summarizes their findings.

Nurse Injury

Table 10-5 lists one study (Stone & Gershon, 2006) of occupational safety outcomes for nurses that included both Magnet to non-Magnet comparisons and PES-NWI comparisons. Findings significantly associated Magnet status with lower rates on all three outcome measures: musculoskeletal injury; blood or body fluid exposure and blood-borne pathogen exposure; and any injury defined as "the summation of all occupational health incident reports" (Stone & Gershon, 2006, p. 242). The study found that more positive organizational climates, measured as a composite PNWE score, were significantly and inversely related to only two of the three measured occupational health outcomes: musculoskeletal injury and any injury.

Patient Outcomes

Magnet to non-Magnet Comparisons

Two studies listed in Table 10-5 compared rates for selected nurse-sensitive indicators between Magnet and non-Magnet organizations. One (Dunton et al., 2007) found that fall rates were 10.3% lower in Magnet organizations but discerned no significant differences between Magnet and non-Magnet organizations for rate of hospital-acquired pressure ulcers. The other (Stone, Mooney-Kane, Larson, Horan et al., 2007) likewise found no association between Magnet status and pressure ulcers; neither did it identify any associations based on Magnet status for central line-associated bloodstream infections, catheter-associated urinary tract infections, or ventilator-associated pneumonia. The results of these studies are summarized in Table 10-6.

PES-NWI Comparisons

Five studies listed in Table 10-5 used PES or PNWE composite or subscale scores to investigate the relationship of Magnet practice environment factors to a number of patient outcomes. As Table 10-6 shows, the results are mixed and often insignificant. Two studies (Manojlovich et al., 2009; Stone, Mooney-Kane, Larson, Horan et al., 2007) found no association between practice environment and either pressure ulcers or ventilator-associated pneumonia. The same two studies demonstrated no link from practice environment to central line-associated bloodstream infection in one case (Manojlovich et al., 2009), and a counterintuitive link in the other (Stone, Mooney-Kane, Larson, Horan et al., 2007). The latter study also found an association between more positive practice environments and lower incidence of catheter-associated urinary tract infections.

Two studies (Aiken et al., 2008; Friese et al., 2008) found significantly lower risks of death and failure to rescue in organizations with better care environments as measured by a PES-NWI composite score. In the first study (Aiken et al., 2008), these findings related to patients who underwent general surgical, orthopedic, or vascular procedures. In the second, surgical oncology patients were studied (Friese et al., 2008). The second study also investigated the relationship between care environment and patient complications and found no association. Two additional studies of patient mortality summarized in Table 10-6 yielded less favorable findings. Using a PNWE composite measure, one study (Stone, Mooney-Kane, Larson, Horan et al., 2007) found no relationship between practice environment and 30-day mortality. Using three PES-NWI subscale measures, the other study (Tourangeau et al., 2006) discovered inconsistent findings across the measures. Lower 30-day mortality rates were related to higher levels of staffing and resource adequacy and lower levels of manager ability as reported by nurses. Nurse reports of collegial nurse–physician relations were not related to mortality.

DISCUSSION

The findings from studies investigating the relationship of Magnet environments with job satisfaction, intent to leave, and quality of care are remarkably consistent and positive. Among the 13 studies that examined job satisfaction or intent to leave or both, only one reported no relationship to working in a Magnet organization (Kovner et al., 2009) and two reported no relationship in some instances but not in others (Chen & Johantgen, 2010; Stone, Larson et al., 2006). For the five studies that examined quality of care, only the study of geriatric care in hospitals (Kim et al., 2009) found no associations or negative associations between some Magnet characteristics and the outcome variable.

Except for the single study of nurse occupational health outcomes (Stone & Gershon, 2006), results were mixed from the three remaining groups of studies reviewed: patient outcome, patient satisfaction, and nurse survey on safety-related topics. Inconsistent findings can result from a variety of factors such as different designs, variability in measures, weak measures,

Table 10-5. Studies With Outcomes Based on Organizational Data: Magnet and Outcome Measures

Article	Magnet Measure(s)	Associated or Dependent Variable(s)
Dunton et al., 2007	Magnet recognition	*Unit data:* Rate of falls Rate of hospital-acquired pressure ulcers
Stone & Gershon, 2006	Magnet recognition PNWE – 7 scales composite	*Incident reports:* Musculoskeletal injury Blood or body fluid exposure and blood-borne pathogen exposure Any injury
Stone, Mooney-Kane, Larson, Horan, et al., 2007 [Med Care]	Magnet recognition PNWE – 7 scales composite	*Infection data:* Central line-associated bloodstream infections Catheter-associated urinary tract infections Ventilator-associated pneumonia *Medicare data:* Decubitus ulcer 30-day mortality
Aiken et al., 2008	PES/NWI – 3 scales composite	*Discharge data:* Failure to rescue 30-day mortality
Friese et al., 2008	PES/NWI – 5 scales composite	*Discharge data:* Patient complications Failure to rescue 30-day mortality
Manojlovich et al., 2009	PES/NWI – 5 scales composite	*Administrative data:* Bloodstream infection associated with central catheter Pressure ulcers Ventilator-associated pneumonia
Tourangeau et al., 2006	NWI-R – 3 scales	*Discharge data:* 30-day mortality

missing variables (variables important to a relationship but omitted from the research), or lack of controls for confounding factors (Hearld et al., 2008; Kazanjian et al., 2005; Unruh, 2008). Quantitative research on practice environments, which began fewer than 20 years ago, is relatively new (Lake, 2007), with varied approaches taken to study it. A drawback of the "diversity of conceptual and methodological approaches used to study the relationship with quality [in health services research] … is an inability to converge on conclusions and generalize about the underlying relationships" (Hearld et al., 2008, p. 261).

Table 10-6. Summary of Results for Studies With Outcomes Based on Organizational Data or Reports

Magnet Measure	Falls	Pressure Ulcers	CLABSI[1]	CAUTI[2]	VAP[3]
Magnet recognition					
Dunton et al., 2007	Negative association	No association	na	na	na
Stone, Mooney-Kane, et al., 2007 [Med Care]	na	No association	No association	No association	No association
PES/PNWE composite					
Manojlovich et al., 2009	na	No association	No association	na	No association
Stone, Mooney-Kane, et al., 2007 [Med Care]	na	No association	Positive association	Negative association	No association

	Patient Complications	Failure to Rescue	30-day Mortality
PES/PNWE composite			
Aiken et al., 2008	na	Negative association	Negative association
Friese et al., 2008	No association	Negative association	Negative association
Stone, Mooney-Kane, et al., 2007 [Med Care]	na	na	No association
PES-NWI subscales			
Tourangeau et al., 2006			
Manager ability	na	na	Positive association
Staffing/ resources	na	na	Negative association
RN-MD relations	na	na	No association

Note: na = Not Applicable.
1. CLABSI = Central line cather-associated blood stream infection.
2. CAUTI = Catheter-associated urinary tract infection.
3. VAP = Ventilator-associated pneumonia.

Mixed and inconsistent findings also reflect the complexity of the research question. The contribution of nursing practice environment factors to patient care outcomes is exceedingly difficult for researchers to isolate in the presence of so many confounding factors. These include patient characteristics, the actions of other healthcare providers, and the multiple, overlapping organizational contexts that exist in hospitals. It is not unusual to have poor patient outcomes despite superior caregiver performance. This is due to the other causal factors at work in the care environment (Flood et al., 2006). The difficulty of the research question suggests caution in interpreting findings from studies such as those summarized in Table 10-6, all of which measure quality from a deficiencies perspective. As Kazanjian et al. (2005) noted, "the methodological challenges inherent in measuring the nursing environment and the complexity of its indirect effect on outcomes mean that evidence as to any association has limitations" (p. 115).

HOW THE RESEARCH HAS PROGRESSED

The previous review in Appendix 10-A identified a need to raise the methodological sophistication of the research on nursing practice environments and outcomes. On the whole, the studies summarized in the current review have done that. More patient care outcome variables were constructed from objective sources or from patient reports than from nurse self-reports. Instead of focusing on single variables or just a few variables, most studies in the current review included many independent and control variables, which implies taking a systems approach by considering "a larger, more interconnected web of organizational dynamics" in the analysis (Hoff et al., 2004, p. 23).

Comparing methods among the studies in the current review also reveals researchers' efforts to refine the measurement of practice environment characteristics. For example, three studies (Manojlovich, 2005; Manojlovich & DeCicco, 2007; Manojlovich et al., 2009) augmented the PES-NWI collegial nurse–physician relations subscale. The team included the communication subscale of the ICU Nurse–Physician Questionnaire in order to add items about openness, accuracy, timeliness, and understanding of the communication that occurs between nurses and physicians (Shortell et al., 1991).[3] On the other hand, Aiken et al. (2008) and Kutney-Lee et al. (2009) excluded two PES-NWI subscales—nurse participation in hospital affairs and staffing and resource adequacy—because they empirically overlapped with other study variables that measured nurse staffing and education.

Finally, compared to the studies reviewed in the appendix to this chapter, recent studies were more likely to be specific to particular nursing specialties or unit types and to apply multivariate analysis techniques. Several of the studies reviewed here used hierarchical analysis or other methods to control for clustering and levels within hospitals.

FUTURE RESEARCH

Reviewing the state of the research about Magnet organizations and nurses' work environments reveals a number of conceptual and methodological issues that need to be thoughtfully considered to move research to the next level. Six issues are addressed here: expanding theoretical frameworks; creating more syntheses of relevant literature; including more direct measures of Magnet characteristics in the research; developing missing and needed measures; conducting more large and robust research studies; and exploring new paradigms to investigate complex environments, such as nursing practice environments in healthcare organizations. An accompanying goal is to facilitate the professional critique that is so vital to moving science forward by always providing clear and complete descriptions of methods, measures, data sources, and results in the research accounts published.

Theoretical Frameworks

Theory is well represented in the studies reviewed here. For example, Manojlovich & Laschinger (2007) have been testing theoretical models of structural empowerment, and the PES-NWI offers theoretical relevance because it contains four theory-based domains identified from the literature on job satisfaction and professional practice (Lake, 2007). Nevertheless, researchers need to extend and strengthen the theoretical frameworks for investigating the effects of nursing practice environments on outcomes (e.g., Lu et al., 2005; Mick & Mark, 2005). There is some broader concern among health services researchers that data availability will drive the research (Hearld et al., 2008). With so many variables affecting outcomes in the care environment, it is more difficult to determine the important relationships without theory to guide the questions. Theory helps to "organize inherently complex and abstract concepts … [it] moves us beyond the 'what' to questions of 'how' and 'why'" (Hearld et al., 2008, p. 271).

Literature Synthesis

The field needs more systematic reviews of the literature to synthesize research on the relationship of the major concepts in the Magnet framework to outcomes for patients, nurses, and organizations. This review has focused exclusively on Magnet recognition or the 16 overlapping subscales of the three NWI-derived tools we encountered in the studies under review. But the Magnet framework represents dozens of variables at multiple levels of abstraction. These include the 14 Forces of Magnetism identified in the original Magnet research (McClure et al., 1983), the five components of the new Magnet Model (chapters in this volume), and the 88 criteria specified in the 2008 *Application Manual: Magnet Recognition Program* (ANCC, 2008). The existing literature may already include adequate measures for many of these concepts. For example, Kazanjian et al. (2005) identified 27 studies of patient mortality and practice environment factors based on Magnet concepts; and Laschinger et al. (2004) represented Structural Empowerment with measures of the access to opportunity, information, support, and resources and the perceptions of formal and informal power that overlap with Magnet characteristics.

Both qualitative and quantitative considerations of the literature are needed. Reviews that provide more detailed synthesis by distinguishing the organizational level of analysis (Hearld et al., 2008; Mitchell & Shortell, 1997) and that classify studies by unit type or nursing specialty would be valuable. This work to synthesize findings from studies that used different methods, different units of analysis, and different levels of aggregation would help to estimate the weight of the evidence that links Magnet environment factors to outcomes.

Direct Measures of Magnet Characteristics

Studies comparing Magnet and non-Magnet organizations have helped to develop an outline of the possible relationships between patient, workforce, or organizational outcomes and more positive practice environments for nurses. However, application for Magnet recognition is voluntary, and many healthcare organizations that have chosen not to apply for Magnet recognition may be providing excellent care from competent nurses in superior work environments. We might think of them as the "virtual" Magnets in research studies that include organizations both with and without Magnet recognition status. Kovner et al. (2009) provided an example of this when they found that Magnet status related to organizational commitment in one analysis, but the relationship disappeared when direct measures of organizational constraints were added back into the model. Hence, the team's suggestion that "future researchers should be cautious when choosing hospitals that do not have Magnet status as comparisons to Magnet hospitals, because the non-Magnet hospitals may be quite similar" (p. 90).

In research, Magnet recognition has stood as a rough proxy for some underlying characteristics of interest that would be better measured directly. This would control for virtual Magnets in the study sample and improve understanding about which practice environment factors influence which outcomes and how. Many of the studies reviewed in this chapter measured Magnet characteristics directly via the PES-NWI or similar instrument. But the new *Magnet Application Manual* specifies at least 88 criteria that define a Magnet environment. Thus, researchers must develop and test many more measures for assessing the degree to which dimensions of Magnet practice environments are present in an organization. For example, if Dunton et al. (2007) found significantly lower fall rates in Magnet organizations, what might we hypothesize as the underlying structure and process characteristics of Magnet environments that work to prevent falls? And what practical, effective tools might we develop to measure them directly?

Measures Development

Researchers must find environmental measures that reflect concepts in the Magnet framework and are logically related to outcomes of interest. Measures of process are notably more difficult to develop than measures of structure. However, except in relation to staffing and professionalization (usually defined as autonomy of the clinical staff), structure–outcome studies have been "plagued with nonsignificant results" (Hearld et al., 2008, p. 265), and process characteristics are likely to be more "proximal indicators of quality" (p. 262). An "objective of hospital quality research" should be to develop "standardized instruments for common process variables such as leadership, culture, and communication [that] might facilitate routine data collection" and eventually lead to making secondary data on hospital processes readily available (p. 276).

Large, Robust Studies

More studies that use longitudinal methods to specify causal connections and mixed methods to supplement quantitative interpretations with qualitative information would be valuable. Multi-level models are particularly important because they account for context when social processes operate at multiple levels of analysis as they do in healthcare organizations. Consider DiPrete and Forristal's (1994) description of the most complicated instances: "Multiple contexts can apply to a given unit. Contexts can be overlapping or nested. They can have fuzzy boundaries or clear ones. Not surprisingly, more complex specifications can introduce formidable methodological difficulties" (p. 333). When multi-level techniques are not applied to the analysis of data that represent patients embedded in units and units embedded in hospitals, researchers can mis-specify relationships (Dunton et al., 2007).

In addition, investigators must conduct more large, adequately powered studies to move science forward and build the knowledge base for practice. Many studies are conducted with samples too small to detect differences and can serve only as pilot work. Although researchers may often state that their study should be replicated with larger samples to determine if pilot results can be generalized to a population, many pilots are never taken to the next level of a fully powered and refined study. More collaborative research is needed in well-designed, large, multi-site studies that can contribute to science and the evidence for practice and care. Investigators must embrace new models to conduct high-quality research if the profession expects to understand the phenomena important to practice and patient care outcomes.

New Paradigms

The basic tradition of research has derived from biomedical and scientific frameworks of mechanism and reductionism, which have been effective for answering some questions. However, conventional traditions are not always a good fit for some of the research areas of interest for nurses. Many nursing activities are nonlinear and complex and may be better understood through a complex dynamic systems approach (Engebretson & Hickey, 2010). Healthcare organizations and nurses' work environments are highly complex and dynamic entities. One new investigatory approach is complexity science. This emerging paradigm is concerned with the interconnections between individual units (called agents) in dynamic, complex, nonlinear systems. Weather forecasting, economics, neuroscience physiology, and organizational behavior are a few examples of areas in which complexity science has been applied.

The following provides a brief description of complexity science and, more specifically, complex adaptive systems. Complexity science is not a single unifying theory, but includes a number of constructs, metaphors, theories, and frameworks that have been applied to health care, social behavior, and organizations. A complex adaptive system (CAS) refers to a special form of complexity science and has been a useful framework for investigating practice environments because it examines the *relationships* among the units, components, or agents rather than just the components themselves (Anderson et al., 2003; Crabtree et al., 2001).

A CAS is a network of individual agents in constant dynamic interactions with each other. It has a high degree of adaptive capacity and the features of self-similarity, complexity, emergence, and self-organization (Zimmerman et al., 1998). A CAS follows simple rules. It has the ability to adapt, which allows the agent or organization to continually modify itself to a changing environment and become a good "fit" by changing the rules of interaction among component agents (Plsek & Greenhalgh, 2001). A CAS has the freedom to act in ways that are not always predictable. Its actions are interconnected so that the action of one part changes the context for other agents (Wilson et al., 2001). Small change can have a big impact on the system, and conversely, big changes in one area may produce little change elsewhere. Control within a CAS is decentralized and dispersed so that leadership can emerge anywhere within a system. Coherent behavior arises from competition and cooperation among the agents (Waldrop, 1992). The process of adaptation in a dynamic environment occurs through learning new rules or behaviors and accumulating new experiences. It allows for creativity and lacks complete predictability. Although similar to systems theory, a big difference is that in systems theory, the whole is equal to the sum of its parts, whereas in complexity science, the whole is different and more than the sum of its parts (Strumberg & Martin, 2009).

Conceptual and Methodological Considerations

How does CAS information apply to research focused on understanding work environments for nurses? First, work and practice environments are complex systems that can be described as social organizations. The many interventions nurses and other agents employ in healthcare organizations have multiple components, some of which are interpersonal and focused on learning. Thus, the interpersonal and learning components are examples of organizational social change. Organizations preparing to apply for Magnet recognition are said to be on the Magnet journey. Along the way, an organization undertakes an in-depth analysis of its structures, processes, and outcomes through a quality improvement lens. The goal is to make changes to meet high standards. These activities change organizations. As the culture changes, embedding Magnet standards is necessary to sustain excellence.

Second, when studying linear, mechanical relationships, it may be useful to employ research designs that follow an observation-intervention-observation methodology, such as in a randomized control design. However, researchers may need other designs to understand the complex work and practice environment in healthcare organizations. Jordon et al. (2010), studying complex healthcare organizations for several years, say that the task of interpreting research observations of healthcare organizations could be improved if researchers regarded each system they study as a CAS with non-linear relationships among diverse learning agents. Research models and methodologies need to match the complexity and dynamics of the CAS. Without such models, it will not be possible to fully understand what makes a healthcare facility outstanding for both nurses and patients.

Third, in randomized controlled trials and other designs with a comparison group, the researcher tries to remove the local cultural details from the design to focus on the variables of interest for purposes of generalization. If one removes the local details about "how" something works, as well as the "what" of context, it will reveal little about the mechanisms or factors that affect generalization (Berwick, 2008). One of the goals of research on work environments is to uncover what makes an outstanding environment so it can be applied to other settings. Berwick goes on to say that studying a few covariates, using stratified designs, or probing for interactions can mitigate this loss, but these are inadequate tools for studying complex, unstable, nonlinear social change.

Fourth, are there methodologies available for research design and statistical analysis using a complexity science approach? Researchers have made progress in addressing methodology and design for investigating complex systems such as healthcare organizations (Anderson & McDaniel, 2008; McDaniel et al., 2009). For example, Bar-Yam (2000) has been instrumental in the development of techniques to study nonlinear dynamics in complex systems. To understand social systems, researchers have combined an ethnographic methodology with agent-based modeling (Agar, 1996). Investigators are using mathematical modeling to understand large-scale, dynamic social systems (Weidlich, 2000). Other methodologies will continue to emerge as researchers determine new ways to study dynamic, complex, nonlinear systems. The Institute of Medicine (2001) noted that approaching health care as a system will be critical to improving quality of care and patient safety. Providers must recognize that *systems* deliver high-quality health care. Researchers will need to use methodologies to help providers understand the relationship of systems to outcomes.

CONCLUSIONS

Due largely to the availability of the PES-NWI, a body of consistent and comparable evidence has been building that shows favorable relationships between Magnet environment characteristics and nurse job satisfaction, nurses' intent to leave, and nurse-perceived quality of care. The PES-NWI is theory-based, valid, reliable, and easy to use (Lake, 2007). Moreover, investigators have successfully tested its validity at both the unit and individual RN level for quality improvement and research purposes (Gajewski et al., 2010). Currently, the PES-NWI does not represent four additional domains that were identified in the literature as theoretically relevant: autonomy, professional development, supportive relationship with peers, and recognition and advancement based on nurse preparation and expertise (Lake, 2007). All are central concepts within the Magnet framework.

If literature reviews identify gaps in available tools, researchers may need to develop new measures to assess the key dimensions defined by Magnet standards. As we have argued here, advancing research on Magnet environments will require several key steps. These include: synthesizing the findings from research on concepts encompassed by the Magnet framework; creating needed measures for concepts not adequately represented in the literature; developing research hypotheses that link specific Magnet characteristics to specific logical outcomes; applying more sophisticated methodologies that can take account of the nested nature of units and subunits within hospitals; and conducting large-scale studies capable of producing generalizable knowledge.

The nursing practice environment contains structural factors and other "modifiable organizational attributes … often termed 'organizational culture' in management studies [that] are key factors for determining hospital performance" (Kazanjian et al., 2005, p. 112). For a variety of reasons, healthcare organizations have been challenged to apply the best available clinical and management knowledge and to implement innovations effectively. Among the remedies the management research literature suggests (Nembhard et al., 2009; Ramanujam & Rousseau, 2006) are several that figure prominently in Magnet Recognition Program expectations: to incorporate Transformational Leadership, develop high-involvement work systems, enhance staff and management competencies, create non-threatening opportunities for innovation adaptation, and, in general, think organizationally. These themes work both individually and collectively to define a research program.

Progress in the quality and quantity of research on nurses' work environments, organizations, and patient outcomes has advanced understanding about their relationships and their contributions to national initiatives for improving patient care quality and safety. The next steps to continue the momentum and gain deeper knowledge of how practice environments influence outcomes are clear. The nursing profession is poised to take on the daunting work of understanding the complexity of practice and care environments.

ENDNOTES

1. Six databases were consistently searched: the National Library of Medicine's PubMed.gov; Cumulative Index of Nursing and Allied Health Literature (CINAHL); Business Source Corporate; Biomedical Reference Collection: Corporate; Education Resource Information Center (ERIC); and SocINDEX.

2. Although safety climate is not typically regarded as an outcome variable, we decided to include the results from the two safety climate studies because of the national concern over patient safety and the work environment of nurses (IOM, 2004).

3. The PES-NWI collegial nurse-physician relations subscale consists of three items: physicians and nurses have good working relationships; a lot of teamwork between nurses and doctors; and functional collaboration (joint practice) between nurses and physicians (Lake, 2002).

REFERENCES

All URLs retrieved September 12, 2010.

Agar, M. H. (1996). *The professional stranger: An informal introduction to ethnography* (2nd ed.). San Diego, CA: Academic Press.

Aiken, L. H. (2002). Superior outcomes for Magnet hospitals: The evidence base. In M. L. McClure & A. S. Hinshaw (Eds.), *Magnet hospitals revisited: Attraction and retention of professional nurses* (pp. 61-81). Washington, DC: American Nurses Publishing.

Aiken, L. H., Clarke, S. P., Sloane, D. M., Lake, E. T., & Cheney, T. (2008). Effects of hospital care environment on patient mortality and nurse outcomes. *Journal of Nursing Administration, 38*(5), 223–229.

Aiken, L. H., & Patrician, P. A. (2000). Measuring organizational traits of hospitals: The revised nursing work index. *Nursing Research, 49*(3), 146–153.

American Nurses Credentialing Center. (2008). *Application manual: Magnet Recognition Program.* Silver Spring, MD: Author.

Anderson, R. A., Issel, L. M., & McDaniel, R. R. (2003). Nursing homes as complex adaptive systems: Relationship between management practice and resident outcomes. *Nursing Research, 52*(1), 12–21.

Anderson, R. A., & McDaniel, R. R. (2008). Taking complexity science seriously: New research, new methods. In C. Lindberg, S. Nash, & C. Lindberg (Eds.), *On the edge: Nursing in the age of complexity* (pp. 73–95). Allentown, NJ: Plexus Institute.

Armstrong, K., Laschinger, H., & Wong, C. (2009). Workplace empowerment and Magnet hospital characteristics as predictors of patient safety climate. *Journal of Nursing Care Quality, 24*(1), 55–62.

Bar-Yam, Y. (Ed.). (2000). *Unifying themes in complex systems: Proceedings of the first international conference on complex systems.* Cambridge, MA: Perseus Books.

Berwick, D. M. (2008). The science of improvement. *Journal of the American Medical Association, 299*(10), 1182–1184.

Chen, Y. M., & Johantgen, M. E. (2010). Magnet hospital attributes in European hospitals: A multilevel model of job satisfaction. *International Journal of Nursing Studies, 47*(8), 1001–1012.

Choi, J., Bakken, S., Larson, E., Du, Y., & Stone, P. W. (2004). Perceived nursing work environment of critical care nurses. *Nursing Research, 53*(6), 370–378.

Clarke, S. P. (2007). Hospital work environments, nurse characteristics, and sharps injuries. *American Journal of Infection Control, 35*(5), 302–309.

Crabtree, B. F., Miller, W. L., & Strange, K. C. (2001). Understanding practice from the ground up. *Journal of Family Practice, 50*(10), 881–887.

DiPrete, T. A., & Forristal, J. D. (1994). Multilevel models: Methods and substance. *Annual Review of Sociology, 20*, 331–357.

Dunton, N., Gajewski, B., Klaus, S., & Pierson, B. (2007). The relationship of nursing workforce characteristics to patient outcomes. *Online Journal of Issues in Nursing, 12*(3). Retrieved from http://www.nursingworld.org/MainMenuCategories/ANAMarketplace/ANAPeriodicals/OJIN/TableofContents/Volume122007/No3Sept07/NursingWorkforceCharacteristics.aspx

Engerbretson, J., & Hickey, J. H. (2010). Complexity science and complex adaptive systems. In J. B. Butts & K. L. Rich (Eds.), *Philosophies and theories in advanced nursing practice.* Sudbury, MA: Jones & Bartlett.

Flood, A. B., Zinn, J. S., & Scott, W. R. (2006). Organizational performance: Managing for efficiency and effectiveness. In S. M. Shortell & A. D. Kaluzny (Eds.), *Healthcare management: Organization design and behavior* (5th ed.), (pp. 415–454). Clifton Park, NY: Thomson Delmar Learning.

Friese, C. R., Lake, E. T., Aiken, L. H., Silber, J. H., & Sochalski, J. (2008). Hospital nurse practice environments and outcomes for surgical oncology patients. *Health Services Research, 43*(4), 1145–1163.

Gajewski, B. J., Boyle, D. K., Miller, P. A., Oberhelman, F., & Dunton, N. (2010). A multilevel confirmatory factor analysis of the practice environment scale: A case study. *Nursing Research, 59*(2), 147–153.

Hearld, L. R., Alexander, J. A., Fraser, I., & Jiang, H. J. (2008). Review: How do hospital organizational structure and processes affect quality of care? A critical review of research methods. *Medical Care Research and Review, 65*(3), 259–299.

Hoff, T., Jameson, L., Hannan, E., & Flink, E. (2004). A review of the literature examining linkages between organizational factors, medical errors, and patient safety. *Medical Care Research and Review, 61*(1), 3-37.

Hughes, L. C., Chang, Y., & Mark, B. A. (2009). Quality and strength of patient safety climate on medical-surgical units. *Health Care Management Review, 34*(1), 19–28.

Institute of Medicine (IOM). (2001). *Crossing the quality chasm: A new health system for the 21st century.* Washington, DC: National Academies Press.

Institute of Medicine (IOM). (2004). *Keeping patients safe: Transforming the work environment of nurses.* Washington, DC: National Academies Press.

Jordon, M., Lanham, H. J., Anderson, R. A., & McDaniel, R. R. (2010). Implications of complex adaptive systems theory for interpreting research about healthcare organizations. *Journal of Evaluation in Clinical Practice, 16*(1), 228–231.

Kazanjian, A., Green, C., Wong, J., & Reid, R. (2005). Effect of the hospital nursing environment on patient mortality: A systematic review. *Journal of Health Services Research & Policy, 10*(2), 111–117.

Kim, H., Capezuti, E., Boltz, M., & Fairchild, S. (2009). The nursing practice environment and nurse-perceived quality of geriatric care in hospitals. *Western Journal of Nursing Research, 31*(4), 480–495.

Kovner, C. T., Brewer, C. S., Green, W., & Fairchild, S. (2009). Understanding new registered nurses' intent to stay at their jobs. *Nursing Economic$, 27*(2), 81–98.

Kramer, M., & Hafner, L. P. (1989). Shared values: Impact on staff nurse job satisfaction and perceived productivity. *Nursing Research, 38*(3), 172–177.

Kutney-Lee, A., McHugh, M. D., Sloane, D. M., Cimiotti, J. P., Flynn, L., Neff, D. F., & Aiken, L. H. (2009). Nursing: A key to patient satisfaction. *Health Affairs, 28*(4), 669–677.

Lacey, S. R., Cox, K. S., Lorfing, K. C., Teasley, S. L., Carroll, C. A., & Sexton, K. (2007). Nursing support, workload, and intent to stay in Magnet, Magnet-aspiring, and non-Magnet hospitals. *Journal of Nursing Administration, 37*(4), 199–205.

Lake, E. T. (2002). Development of the practice environment scale of the nursing work index. *Research in Nursing & Health, 25*(3), 176–188.

Lake, E. T. (2007). The nursing practice environment: Measurement and evidence. *Medical Care Research and Review, 64*(2 Suppl), 104S–122S.

Laschinger, H. K. S. (2008). Effect of empowerment on professional practice environments, work satisfaction, and patient care quality: Further testing the nursing worklife model. *Journal of Nursing Care Quality, 23*(4), 322–330.

Laschinger, H. K. S., Almost, J., & Tuer-Hodes, D. (2003). Workplace empowerment and Magnet hospital characteristics: Making the link. *Journal of Nursing Administration, 33*(7-8), 410-422.

Laschinger, H. K. S., Finegan, J. E., Shamian, J., & Wilk, P. (2004). A longitudinal analysis of the impact of workplace empowerment on work satisfaction. *Journal of Organizational Behavior, 25*(4), 527–545.

Lu, H., While, A. E., & Barriball, K. L. (2005). Job satisfaction among nurses: A literature review. *International Journal of Nursing Studies, 42*(2), 211–227.

Lundmark, V. (2008). Magnet environments for professional nursing practice. In R. G. Hughes (Ed.), *Patient safety and quality: An evidence-based handbook for nurses.* AHRQ Publication No. 08-0043. Retrieved from http://www.ahrq.gov/qual/nurseshdbk/

Manojlovich, M. (2005). Linking the practice environment to nurses' job satisfaction through nurse–physician communication. *Journal of Nursing Scholarship, 37*(4), 367–373.

Manojlovich, M., Antonakos, C. L., & Ronis, D. L. (2009). Intensive care units, communication between nurses and physicians, and patients' outcomes. *American Journal of Critical Care, 18*(1), 21–30.

Manojlovich, M., & DeCicco, B. (2007). Healthy work environments, nurse–physician communication, and patients' outcomes. *American Journal of Critical Care, 16*(6), 536–543.

Manojlovich, M., & Laschinger, H. (2007). The nursing worklife model: Extending and refining a new theory. *Journal of Nursing Management, 15*(3), 256–263.

McClure, M. L., Poulin, M. A., Sovie, M. D., & Wandell, M. A. (1983). *Magnet hospitals: Attraction and retention of professional nurses.* Kansas City, MO: American Nurses Association.

McDaniel, R. R., Lanham, H. J., & Anderson, R. A. (2009). Implications of complex adaptive systems theory for the design of research on health care organizations. *Health Care Management Review, 34*(3), 191–199.

McKeon, L. M., Oswaks, J. D., & Cunningham, P. D. (2006). Safeguarding patients: Complexity science, high-reliability organizations, and implications for team training in healthcare. *Clinical Nurse Specialist, 20*(6), 298–304.

Mick, S. S., & Mark, B. A. (2005). The contribution of organization theory to nursing health services research. *Nursing Outlook, 53*(6), 317–323.

Mitchell, P. H., & Shortell, S. M. (1997). Adverse outcomes and variations in organization of care delivery. *Medical Care, 35*(11 Suppl), NS19–32.

National Quality Forum. (2004). *National voluntary consensus standards for nursing-sensitive care: An initial performance measure set—A consensus report.* Washington, DC: National Quality Forum.

Nembhard, I. M., Alexander, J. A., Hoff, T. J., & Ramanujam, R. (2009). Why does the quality of health care continue to lag? Insights from management research. *Journal of Organizational Behavior, 23*(1), 24–42.

Plsek, P. E., & Greenhalgh, T. (2001). Complexity science: The challenge of complexity in health care. *British Medical Journal, 323*(7313), 625–628.

Ramanujam, R., & Rousseau, D. M. (2006). The challenges are organizational not just clinical. *Journal of Organizational Behavior, 27*(7), 811–827.

Schmalenberg, C., & Kramer, M. (2008). Essentials of a productive nurse work environment. *Nursing Research, 57*(1), 2–13.

Seago, J. A. (2008). Unit characteristics and patient satisfaction. *Policy, Politics, & Nursing Practice, 9*(4), 230–240.

Shortell, S. M., Rousseau, D. M., Gillies, R. R., Devers, K. J., & Simons, T. L. (1991). Organizational assessment in intensive care units (ICUs): Construct development, reliability, and validity of the ICU nurse–physician questionnaire. *Medical Care, 29*(8), 709–726.

Siu, H., Laschinger, H. K. S., & Finegan, J. (2008). Nursing professional practice environments: Setting the stage for constructive conflict resolution and work effectiveness. *Journal of Nursing Administration, 38*(5), 250–257.

Stone, P. W., & Gershon, R. R. (2006). Nurse work environments and occupational safety in intensive care units. *Policy, Politics, & Nursing Practice, 7*(4), 240–247.

Stone, P. W., Larson, E. L., Mooney-Kane, C., Smolowitz, J., Lin, S. X., & Dick, A. W. (2006). Organizational climate and intensive care unit nurses' intention to leave. *Critical Care Medicine, 34*(7), 1907–1912.

Stone, P. W., Mooney-Kane, C., Larson, E. L., Horan, T., Glance, L. G., Zwanziger, J., & Dick, A. W. (2007). Nurse working conditions and patient safety outcomes. *Medical Care, 45*(6), 571–578.

Stone, P. W., Mooney-Kane, C., Larson, E. L., Pastor, D. K., Zwanziger, J., & Dick, A. W. (2007). Nurse working conditions, organizational climate, and intent to leave in ICUs: An instrumental variable approach. *Health Services Research, 42*(3, Pt. 1), 1085–1104.

Strumberg, J. P., & Martin, C. M. (2009). Complexity and health—Yesterday's traditions, tomorrow's future. *Journal of Evaluation in Clinical Practice, 15*(3), 543–548.

Tourangeau, A. E., Doran, D. M., Hall, L. M., Pallas, L. O., Pringle, D., Tu, J. V., & Cranley, L. A. (2006). Impact of hospital nursing care on 30-day mortality for acute medical patients. *Journal of Advanced Nursing, 57*(1), 32–44.

Ulrich, B. T., Buerhaus, P. I., Donelan, K., Norman, L., & Dittus, R. (2007). Magnet status and registered nurse views of the work environment and nursing as a career. *Journal of Nursing Administration, 37*(5), 212–220.

Ulrich, B. T., Woods, D., Hart, K. A., Lavandero, R., Leggett, J., & Taylor, D. (2007). Critical care nurses' work environments: Value of excellence in beacon units and Magnet organizations. *Critical Care Nurse, 27*(3), 68–77.

Unruh, L. (2008). Nurse staffing and patient, nurse, and financial outcomes. *American Journal of Nursing, 108*(1), 62–71.

Wade, G. H., Osgood, B., Avino, K., Bucher, G., Bucher, L., Foraker, T., French, D., & Sirkowski, C. (2008). Influence of organizational characteristics and caring attributes of managers on nurses' job enjoyment. *Journal of Advanced Nursing, 64*(4), 344–353.

Waldrop, M. M. (1992). *Complexity: The emerging science at the edge of order and chaos.* New York, NY: Simon & Schuster.

Weidlich, W. (2000). *Sociodynamics: A systematic approach to mathematical modeling in the social sciences.* Mineola, NY: Dover Publications.

Wilson, T., Holt, T., & Greenhalgh, T. (2001). Complexity science: Complexity and clinical care. *British Medical Journal, 323*(7314), 685–688.

Zimmerman, B., Lindberg, C., & Plsek, P. (1998). *Edgeware: Lessons from complexity science for healthcare leaders.* Bordentown, NJ: Plexus Press.

Appendix to Chapter 10

MAGNET ENVIRONMENTS FOR PROFESSIONAL NURSING PRACTICE

The systematic review contained in this appendix was conducted by this chapter's first author in 2006 and published in an Agency for Healthcare Research and Quality (AHRQ) handbook in 2008. That review encompassed 31 research articles that were published from 1987 to 2006 and that both reported results from primary or secondary data analysis and included nurse or patient outcome variables. It is included here to lend greater context to the new material in this chapter. The literature review presented in the chapter extends the review reported in this appendix.

Source: V. A. Lundmark, (2008). Originally published as Chapter 46 in *Patient Safety and Quality: An Evidence-Based Handbook for Nurses* (AHRQ Publication No. 08-0043). Agency for Healthcare Research and Quality, Rockville, MD.

Chapter 46. Magnet Environments for Professional Nursing Practice

Vicki A. Lundmark

Background

In hospital settings, nurses fulfill two roles. Based upon expert knowledge, nurses provide care to the ill or prevent illness. Nurses also maintain and manage the environment surrounding the delivery of care, which has increasingly involved coordinating the care activities provided by other health care providers. Of three reports published since the year 2000 by the Institute of Medicine,[1-3] the 2004 report on patient safety was the first to emphasize the connection between nursing, patient safety, and quality of care. The report specifically noted the importance of organizational management practices, strong nursing leadership, and adequate nurse staffing for providing a safe care environment. The report also noted how frequently the patient safety practices identified by the literature "were the same as those recommended by organizations studying the nursing shortage, worker safety, and patient satisfaction"[3] (p. 317).

While it seems logical to assume that safe and effective patient care depends on the presence of "an organizational context that enables the best performance from each health professional"[4] (p. 186), remarkably little knowledge has accumulated about how the organization and delivery of nursing services influences patient outcomes. One explanation for this situation is that health services research so firmly turned its focus to organization/environment and organization/market questions following the rise of health economics and health maintenance organizations (HMOs) in the 1970s that it was caught somewhat unprepared when quality issues began to emerge in the latter part of the 1990s. As a result, few conceptual tools exist "to address the heart of quality concerns: the internal work processes and arrangements inside health care organizations . . . that contribute to variations in quality"[5] (p. 318).

Another limiting factor has been the inherent challenges of measuring organizational practice environments and the complexity of nursing's effects on patient outcomes. Improved theoretical frameworks and greater methodological rigor will be needed to guide and advance the nursing research on patient outcomes.[6, 7] Nursing research has already been leading the way in this effort, which may not be surprising given the deep knowledge nurses have of the internal workings of health care organizations.[5]

The magnet hospital concept, originating from a groundbreaking study in the early 1980s[8] that sought to explain instances of successful nurse recruitment and retention during a severe nurse shortage, provides one framework for specifying the organizational and practice environment conditions that support and facilitate nursing excellence. The purpose of this chapter is to summarize the magnet research evidence related to nurse or patient outcomes.

Magnet Hospitals and the Attraction and Retention of Professional Nurses

The original magnet study began in 1981 when the American Academy of Nursing appointed a task force to investigate the factors impeding or facilitating professional nursing practice in hospitals. The four researchers on the task force were working from the knowledge that despite a nursing shortage for a large number of hospitals, a certain number "had succeeded in creating nursing practice organizations that serve as 'magnets' for professional nurses; that is, they are able to attract and retain a staff of well-qualified nurses and are therefore consistently able to provide quality care"[8] (p. 2). Therefore, the research goal was set to explore the factors associated with success in attracting and retaining professional nurses.

Through an extensive nominating process, 41 hospitals from across the country were selected to participate in the study based upon their known reputations as being good places for nurses to work and the evidence they submitted to document a relatively low nurse turnover rate.[9] Subsequently, a series of group interviews was held with representatives from each hospital. Two interviews were conducted in each of eight geographically dispersed locations. In the morning, one of the task force researchers interviewed the chief nurse executives from the participating hospitals in that area. Then, in the afternoon, a second group interview session was held with staff nurses. Each staff nurse who participated in the interviews was selected by his or her chief nurse executive.

Based upon their analysis of this interview data, the task force researchers identified and defined a set of characteristics that seemed to account for the success the 41 reputational magnet hospitals had enjoyed in attracting and keeping a staff of well-qualified nurses at a time when other hospitals around them were not able to do so. The labels given to these characteristics, which have come to be known as the forces of magnetism, are listed below in Table 1. Many of the insights they embody have a long history of study within the sociological literature related to organizational performance, leadership, worker autonomy and motivation, decentralized or participative management, work design, coordination and communication, effective groups and teams, and organizational innovation and change.[10]

Table 1. The Magnet Characteristics of a Professional Practice Environment

Forces of Magnetism 1983 (McClure)[8]	Forces of Magnetism 2005 (ANCC)[11]
Administration	
Quality of leadership	1. Quality of nursing leadership
Organizational structure	2. Organizational structure
Management style	3. Management style
Staffing	4. Personnel policies and programs
Personnel policies and programs	[staffing embedded in #4]
Professional practice	
Professional practice models	5. Professional models of care
Quality of care	6. Quality of care
Quality assurance	7. Quality improvement
Consultation and resources	8. Consultation and resources
Autonomy	9. Autonomy
Community and the hospital	10. Community and the hospital
Nurses as teachers	11. Nurses as teachers
Image of nursing	12. Image of nursing
Nurse-physician relationships	13. Interdisciplinary relationships
Professional development	
Orientation	14. Professional development [original
In-service and continuing education	subgroups embedded]
Formal education	
Career development	

Note: Order shown in the left column has been slightly rearranged for ease of comparison.

The relationship of a magnet environment to quality was recently described by one of the original task force researchers. Looking back on the original magnet study more than 20 years later, McClure wrote[12] (p. 199),

> We found that all these settings had a commonality: their corporate cultures were totally supportive of nursing and of quality patient care. What we learned was that this culture permeated the entire institution. It was palpable and it seemed to be almost a part of the bricks and mortar. Simply stated, these were good places for all employees to work (not just nurses) and these were good places for patients to receive care. The goal of quality was not only stated in the mission of these institutions but it was lived on a daily basis.

The Magnet Recognition Program® of the American Nurses Credentialing Center (ANCC)*

In the early 1990s, the American Nurses Association (ANA) initiated a pilot project to develop an evaluation program based upon the conceptual framework identified by the 1983 magnet research. The program's infrastructure was established within the newly incorporated American Nurses Credentialing Center of the ANA, and the first facility to receive Magnet recognition was named in 1994.[11] Interest in Magnet™ has been increasingly accelerating. While only about 225 organizations have achieved Magnet recognition since the program's inception, nearly two-thirds of them did so within the last 3 years, and the applicant list continues to expand.

Applicants for Magnet recognition undergo a lengthy and comprehensive appraisal process[13] to demonstrate that they have met the criteria for all of the forces of magnetism shown in the right column of Table 1. Currently, documentation or sources of evidence are required in support of 164 topics.[11] Organizations that receive high scores on written documentation move to the site-visit stage of the appraisal and a period of public comment. The philosophy of the program is that nurses function at their peak when a Magnet environment is fully expressed and embedded throughout the health care organization, wherever nursing is practiced. Magnet organizations submit annual reports and must reapply every 4 years to maintain their recognition.

In the context of a rapidly evolving health care system, ANCC has the responsibility as a credentialing body to continuously refine and improve the criteria it uses for Magnet recognition in order to "separate true magnets from those that simply want to achieve the recognition"[14] (p. 123). ANCC does so by evaluating new information from multiple sources, the scholarly research literature, expert groups convened to deliberate specific issues, and feedback from Magnet facilities and appraisers, particularly in relation to identifying effective and innovative practices.

Continuity between the original magnet research and ANCC's Magnet program is provided by the conceptual framework for the forces of magnetism. Little has changed in the essential definitions for the forces except that ANCC has revised them to reflect contemporary hospital settings and elaborated under each force a set of required documentation for applicants to submit and appraisers to evaluate. Beginning in 2005, however, an important change appeared in the

---

* The Magnet Recognition Program® and ANCC Magnet Recognition® names and logos are registered trademarks of the American Nurses Credentialing Center. Magnet™ is a trademark of the American Nurses Credentialing Center. Magnet is capitalized in this chapter when it refers to the ANCC Magnet Recognition Program or to organizations that have been designated Magnet by the Magnet Recognition Program.

Magnet application process. Whereas previous application manuals had itemized evidence requirements according to ANA's *Scope and Standards for Nurse Administrators*,[15] the new manual version[11] reorganized the criteria into the framework of the forces of magnetism. This transition should help to clarify the correspondence between the elements ANCC's Magnet program evaluates in its appraisal process and the magnet characteristics that nursing and health services researchers study.

Reviewing the Evidence

Research studies were retrieved for this review by searching PubMed® and CINAHL® for articles referencing magnet or magnetism in the title or abstract. Two inclusion criteria were used. (More details can be found below, in "Search Strategy.") The articles had to (a) report findings from analyses of primary or secondary data, and (b) investigate relationships between magnet variables and nurse or patient outcomes. Nurse outcomes of interest were job satisfaction, burnout, and intention to leave[16, 17] or similar variables such as mental health. Nurse perceptions of patient care quality has been a frequently used measure in the magnet-related survey research, and one study used nurse perceptions of safety climate as the dependent variable. But studies that included patient outcome variables measured from other sources were seldom found, although patient mortality and patient satisfaction are represented in the evidence tables.

Limitations of the Research

Overwhelmingly, the magnet research has been dominated by cross-sectional survey studies with convenience samples of organizations and staff nurse respondents. The basic approaches used to capture magnet environments in the research have been to include organizations from the 1983 magnet study or with ANCC Magnet recognition in the hospital sample or to administer survey scales believed to measure magnet characteristics, traits, or factors. Usually, but not always, these approaches have been used in combination. Analyses have typically been limited to simple comparisons of survey items or subscale results between two groups.

With few exceptions, the majority of this research has suffered from two major limitations: biased sampling at both the organizational and respondent level; and a scarcity of comprehensive, valid, and reliable measures for assessing the level of magnet characteristics present in any setting. Unless magnet characteristics are measured adequately across the organizations participating in a study, the degree to which their presence differs between the comparison groups cannot be assessed. Because the organizations that have attained ANCC Magnet recognition constitute a voluntary sample, it is possible that high levels of some or many magnet characteristics may also exist in other organizations that have not chosen to apply for the recognition.

Overwhelmingly, the survey scales most frequently used to measure magnet characteristics have all derived from the Nursing Work Index (NWI). Because these scales have dominated the magnet research, it is important to understand how they are constituted and how they have evolved over time. The first version of the NWI was designed to inclusively and comprehensively reflect the findings of the 1983 magnet research study.[18] It was intended to measure four variables: work values related to staff nurse job satisfaction, work values related to perceived productivity, staff nurse job satisfaction, and perceived productivity (the perception of an environment conducive to quality nursing care). Content validity for the instrument was assured by having three of the four original magnet researchers review it for inclusiveness.[19] The NWI consisted of 65 items and asked respondents to make three Likert-scale judgments on each item.

Aiken[20] subsequently adapted the NWI to measure only organizational features by dropping the judgment statements related to job satisfaction and perceived productivity. Compared to the NWI, the NWI-Revised (NWI-R) contained fewer items, but otherwise remained the same except that one item was modified and two more were added. Four NWI-R subscales were conceptually derived from an item subset.[21]

Two of the NWI-R subscale domains, nurse autonomy and nurse-physician relationships, are readily recognizable in comparison to the forces of magnetism listed in Table 1. The other two domains, organizational support and control over nursing practice, are represented by sets of items that could be classified across several forces of magnetism. Control over nursing practice is defined as organizational autonomy or the freedom to take the initiative in shaping unit and institutional policies for patient care. Hinshaw[22] described clinical autonomy and organizational autonomy as interactive concepts. Both types of autonomy were evident in the findings from the original magnet study.[8, 23]

Since the NWI-R was developed nearly a decade before any subsequent NWI-derived scale versions appeared, the NWI-R has been the most frequently used measure of magnet characteristics in magnet research. An advantage of this fact has been the ability to compare findings across studies. A disadvantage may have been the formation of a wide impression that the magnet hospital concept is more circumscribed than it actually is. In the literature reviewed here, the phrase most frequently used to introduce the magnet concept to readers directly cites the NWI-R subscales; magnet is said to describe hospitals where nurses have greater autonomy, control over nursing practice, and good nurse-physician relationships. Given nursing's history as a subordinated profession,[24] one can understand that these three dimensions of the magnet concept attracted the most initial attention.

In the last 5 years, three additional versions of the NWI have appeared. Except for minor changes in wording, all use items from the NWI or the NWI-R as originally written. However, each version consists of different, empirically derived scale or subscale formations. Lake[25] created the 31-item Practice Environment Scale of the NWI (PES/NWI) with five subscales and an overarching composite scale. Estabrooks and colleagues[26] created a single-factor, 26-item scale called the Practice Environment Index (PEI). Choi and colleagues[27] created the Perceived Nursing Work Environment scale (PNWE)[†] with 42 items and 7 subscales. Neither the PEI nor the PNWE measures appear in the studies reviewed here.

Research Evidence

The evidence tables in this chapter are divided into three parts. Evidence Table 1 covers the early research period and itemizes studies conducted with hospitals from the group of 41 reputational magnets that participated in the 1983 study. Evidence Table 2 includes studies that compared health care organizations with and without designation as ANCC-recognized Magnets. Finally, Evidence Table 3 itemizes studies that investigated the relationship of various magnet

[†] Subscales for the PNWE are labeled professional practice, staffing and resource adequacy, nurse management, nursing process, nurse-physician collaboration, nurse competence, and positive scheduling climate.

characteristics to outcomes. Insofar as possible, the evidence tables are arranged in chronological order to illustrate how magnet research has progressed since the concept of a magnet environment first appeared in the literature in the 1980s. In addition, each row or panel in the tables represents a single data collection event. If multiple articles were generated from a single data collection effort, they are cited together in the same panel of the table. The purpose of this arrangement is to present a clearer picture of the body of evidence as a whole, revealing that the total number of data sources (with their associated measures and methods) that have constituted the magnet research since 1983 is relatively small. In addition, this arrangement draws attention to which articles are better read as a set by anyone wishing to understand the research in detail. Methodological information related to a single data collection effort can sometimes be scattered across multiple publications.

Evidence Table 1 includes two of the most compelling studies to have come out of the magnet literature, those initiated by Aiken and her colleagues[28-35] within a decade of the publication of the original magnet study. For the Medicare mortality study[28], magnet characteristics were not directly measured. However, the use of risk adjustment techniques for predicted mortality and multivariate matched sampling methods to control for factors that might affect mortality provided strong support for concluding that the set of reputational magnet hospitals was uniquely different as a group. As Aiken has summarized it, these "findings suggest that the same factors that lead hospitals to be identified as effective from the standpoint of the organization of nursing care are associated with lower mortality"[20] (p. 72).

Guided by a conceptual framework originating in the sociology of organizations and professions,[20] the second compelling study[29-35] was formulated to examine how certain modifications to the organization of nursing in hospitals introduced by the AIDS epidemic affected patient and nurse outcomes. The AIDS epidemic in combination with high nurse vacancy rates caused a number of urban hospitals to grant "unusual discretion to nurses to redesign general medical units into dedicated AIDS units"[20] (p. 63). Since the comparison group of hospitals for this study included two reputational magnet hospitals and a third hospital believed to be magnet-comparable, the researchers were able to discern that many of the same positive results achieved in dedicated AIDS units could apparently be attained by making changes at the organizational level. Magnet characteristics (as measured by the NWI-R subscales) were associated with significantly better outcomes for nurse safety, job burnout, patient satisfaction, and mortality 30 days from admission.

The studies shown in Evidence Table 2 consistently display positive results relating magnet characteristics (as measured by the NWI-R or PES/NWI subscales) to nurse job satisfaction, burnout, intention to leave, and perceived quality of care. The exception to this finding is the mixed results shown for the nurse-physician relationship subscale. Havens's[36] study with chief nurse executives found higher levels on the NWI-R subscales to be associated with reports of higher patient care quality, less recruitment difficulty, and fewer patient/family complaints. The studies shown in the first two rows of Evidence Table 2, which demonstrated more favorable results for the ANCC Magnet group compared to the reputational magnet group, also supported the view expressed by McClure and Hinshaw that magnet status "is not a permanent institutional characteristic but rather one that requires constant nurturing"[14] (p. 119).

Evidence Table 3 lists three studies that explored the degree to which magnet characteristics could be found in hospitals outside the United States or in nonhospital settings. Thomas-Hawkins and colleagues[37] and Smith, Tallman, and Kelly[38] found that some magnet characteristics linked significantly to intentions to leave in freestanding dialysis units and to job satisfaction in rural

Canadian hospitals, respectively. Rondeau and Wagar[39] found significant associations between magnet characteristics and resident satisfaction and nurse satisfaction, turnover, and vacancy rates in long-term care organizations in western Canada.

The remaining studies shown in Evidence Table 3 are important for a number of reasons. Using multiple measures, a variety of samples and respondent groups, and more powerful analyses, Laschinger and her colleagues[40-44] have been testing a theoretical model linking structural empowerment and magnet characteristics (as measured by the NWI-R or PES/NWI) to nurse and patient outcomes with variables such as trust and burnout posited as mediators. The empowerment dimensions being measured—perceptions of formal and informal power and access to opportunity, information, support, and resources—also appear to overlay some descriptions of magnet characteristics from the original 1983 research. By testing relationships with a set of theoretically selected variables and multivariate statistical methods, the studies of Laschinger and colleagues have been progressively building knowledge about how factors in the complex nursing practice environment interact with each other to affect outcomes.

The work that will be required to explicate how the organization and delivery of nursing services functions as a mechanism to improve patient safety and the quality of care has only just begun. The literature review conducted by Lundstrom and colleagues[45] found a number of studies that start to suggest the mechanisms by which organizational and work environment factors influence worker performance and ultimately patient outcomes. However, the authors also noted, "What we do know about changes in organization and structure of hospitals and the potential for those changes to affect patient outcomes pales by comparison to what we do not know"[45] (p. 103).

Reviewing the magnet research presented in this chapter leads to similar conclusions. The evidence almost uniformly shows consistent positive relations between job satisfaction or nurse-assessed quality of care and the magnet characteristics measured by subscales of the NWI-R or PES/NWI. But the connections from those results based on staff nurse surveys to patient outcomes measured objectively by other means have seldom been studied.

In a recent systematic review of the hospital nursing environment's effect on patient mortality, Kazanjian and colleagues[6] found associations between unfavorable environment attributes and higher patient mortality rates in 19 of 27 studies. However, other studies of the same attributes showed contrary or neutral results. Too much variability existed in measures, settings, and methodological rigor across studies to permit any pooling of results. The authors concluded it would be difficult to determine "how to design optimal practice settings until mechanisms linking practice environment to outcomes are better understood"[6] (p. 111).

Evidence-Based Practice Implications

The magnet framework outlined in Table 1 specifies a set of factors important for establishing positive work environments that support professional nursing practice. As the evidence reviewed in this chapter shows, few studies have explored the relationship of magnet characteristics to patient outcomes. Since the associations found were consistently positive, this constitutes a promising body of work, but one that is just beginning to emerge. In contrast, more evidence has accumulated to demonstrate links between magnet characteristics or Magnet recognition and favorable outcomes for nurses such as lower burnout, higher satisfaction, and fewer reports of intentions to leave. The practice implications suggested by these findings have been delineated in detail by the Institute of Medicine's 2004 report on patient safety, which

Patient Safety and Quality: An Evidence-Based Handbook for Nurses

included a comprehensive review of the research that clarifies how nurse outcomes reflect and interact with working conditions to affect patient safety and quality.[3]

Keeping Patients Safe: Transforming the Work Environment of Nurses cited conditions in the work environments of nurses as "the primary sources" of threats to patient safety that "must be addressed if patient safety is to be improved"[3] (p. 47). The report presented a series of recommendations for improving leadership, management, and organizational support practices that emphasizes the increased participation of employees in work design, problem-solving, and organizational decisionmaking as a "key ingredient to successful organizational change"[3] (p. 260). The report noted that high involvement in decisionmaking for nurses "has been studied under a number of constructs, including shared governance, nursing empowerment, control over nursing practice, and clinical autonomy"[3] (p. 122).

In keeping with the realization that threats to patient safety result from complex causes,[2] *Keeping Patients Safe* identified a multifactor approach to creating favorable work environments for nurses. Many of the strategies and goals described in the report correspond to the descriptions of magnet environments initially provided by McClure and colleagues[8] and currently elaborated for contemporary settings in the appraisal criteria for Magnet recognition.[11] For example, of the 27 goals the report listed as "Necessary Patient Safeguards in the Work Environment of Nurses"[3] (p. 16–17), 20 are addressed by the current evidence requirements for Magnet recognition.[11] The multidimensionality of the magnet framework reflects the highly complex, variable, multilevel, and multifaceted nature of nursing practice environments, but it also poses measurement challenges for researchers interested in studying the influence of magnet environments on outcomes.

Research Implications

Mick and Mark[5] have argued that while nursing research has contributed substantially to the knowledge about how internal structures and work processes relate to patient safety and quality outcomes in health care organizations, there is a compelling need to improve the methodological sophistication of the research and to expand the theoretical frameworks that guide it. Many of the suggestions they make for doing so are echoed in the research implications generated by this review. Greater attention needs to be paid to addressing sampling bias issues, improving critical measures, collecting objective data from sources other than nurse self-reports, and designing multilevel and longitudinal studies. As Table 1 reveals, the conceptual definition of a magnet environment encompasses many fields and disciplines from which theoretical insights may be borrowed and tested.

Taking better account of multiple organizational perspectives and hierarchical levels in the research will build knowledge about how the relationships between magnet characteristics and patient outcomes differ by role or practice location. For example, Laschinger, Almost, and Tuer-Hodes[41] found that magnet characteristics and empowerment related differently to each other and to job satisfaction for nurse practitioners than for staff nurses, and Friese's[46] results differed significantly on some magnet characteristics only for oncology nurses. Distinguishing unit locations may be particularly important. Mick and Mark have claimed that "it is the exploration of work structures and processes at the nursing unit level that is contributing to the lion's share of advancing knowledge about what does and does not have an impact on patient and organizational outcomes"[5] (p. 319).

Finally, while the NWI-R and later versions of the NWI have yielded a wealth of useful data, questions have also been raised as to the measurement adequacy of at least three of them.[47] Variable, unpredictable, contextually sensitive, and multifaceted,[25, 47] "the nursing practice environment is a complex construct to conceptualize and measure"[25] (p. 177). Yet developing, improving, and refining measures to reliably capture all of the factors of a magnet environment may be the most important next step.

Conclusion

The magnet concept defines a framework for facilitating the professional practice of nursing that has demonstrated effectiveness in attracting nurses and shows promise for contributing to optimal patient outcomes. There is a compelling need to improve the measures and methods used to research magnet characteristics and environments before the links that connect organizational context to nurse and patient outcomes can be sufficiently understood.

Search Strategy

A series of searches was carried out in October 2006 using the National Library of Medicine's PubMed database and the Cumulative Index of Nursing and Allied Health Literature (CINAHL) database. Several search terms and phrases including the word "magnet" or "magnetism" were tested in both cases. The most effective were "magnet[Title/abstract] and nursing[Title/abstract]" in PubMed and "magnet" in [TI Title] OR "magnet" in [AB Abstract or Author-Supplied Abstract] with advanced search in CINAHL. Supplementary backup searches were also performed substituting the word "magnetism" for "magnet" in CINAHL and the word "hospitals" for "nursing" in PubMed. The PubMed searches yielded 134 unique titles to review. Cross-checking the CINAHL results against the PubMed lists yielded two additional titles.

The overwhelming majority of articles identified by these searches fell into editorial, interpretive, or narrative categories—especially narratives describing how an individual organization prepared for or achieved ANCC Magnet recognition. If an abstract was ambiguous about whether the article reported results from a primary or secondary data analysis, the article itself was retrieved in order to make a determination. The article by Laschinger and Leiter[44] was previously known and not identified by the search strategy.

Author Affiliations

Vicki A. Lundmark, Ph.D., director, research, American Nurses Credentialing Center. E-mail: Vicki.lundmark@ana.org.

References

1. Institute of Medicine. To err is human: building a safer health system. Washington, DC: National Academies Press; 2000.

2. Institute of Medicine. Crossing the quality chasm. Washington, DC: National Academies Press; 2001.

3. Institute of Medicine. Keeping patients safe: transforming the work environment of nurses. Washington, DC: National Academies Press; 2004.

4. Aiken LH. Improving quality through nursing. In: Mechanic D, Rogut LB, Colby DC, et al., eds. Policy challenges in modern health care. New Brunswick, NJ: Rutgers University Press; 2005. p. 177-88.

5. Mick SS, Mark BA. The contribution of organization theory to nursing health services research. Nurs Outlook 2005 Nov-Dec; 53:317-23.

6. Kazanjian A, Green C. Wong J, et al. Effect of the hospital nursing environment on patient mortality: a systematic review. J Health Serv Res Policy 2005 Apr;10:111-7.

7. White P, McGillis Hall L. Patient safety outcomes. In: Doran DM, eds. Nursing-sensitive outcomes: state of the science. Sudbury, MA: Jones and Bartlett Publishers; 2003. p. 211-42.

8. McClure ML, Poulin MA, Sovie MD, et al. Magnet hospitals: attraction and retention of professional nurses. Kansas City, MO: American Nurses' Association; 1983.

9. McClure ML, Poulin MA, Sovie MD, et al. Magnet hospitals: attraction and retention of professional nurses (the original study). In: McClure ML, Hinshaw AS, eds. Magnet hospitals revisited: attraction and retention of professional nurses. Washington, DC: American Nurses Publishing; 2002: p. 1-24.

10. Shortell SM, Kaluzny AD. Health care management: organization design and behavior. 5th ed. Clifton Park, NY: Thomson Delmar Learning; 2006.

11. American Nurses Credentialing Center. Magnet Recognition Program: Application Manual 2005. Silver Spring, MD: American Nurses Credentialing Center; 2004.

12. McClure ML. Magnet hospitals: insights and issues. Nurs Adm Q 2005 Jul-Sep;29(3):198-201.

13. Lundmark VA, Hickey JV. The Magnet recognition program: understanding the appraisal process. J Nurs Care Qual 2006 Oct-Dec; 21:290-4.

14. McClure ML, Hinshaw AS. The future of magnet hospital. In: McClure ML, Hinshaw AS, eds. Magnet hospitals revisited: attraction and retention of professional nurses. Washington, DC: American Nurses Publishing; 2002. p. 117-127.

15. American Nurses Association (ANA). Scope and standards for nurse administrators. 2nd ed. Washington, DC: Nursesbooks.org; 2004.

16. Mark BA, Salyer J, Wan TT. Professional nursing practice: impact on organizational and patient outcomes. J Nurs Adm 2003 Apr; 33:224-34.

17. Stone P, Pastor DK, Harrison MI. Organizational climate: implications for the home healthcare workforce. J Healthc Qual 2006 Jan-Feb; 28:4-11.

18. Kramer M, Schmalenberg CE. Best quality patient care: a historical perspective on Magnet hospitals. Nurs Adm Q 2005 Jul-Sep;29:275-87

19. Kramer M, Hafner LP. Shared values: impact on staff nurse job satisfaction and perceived productivity. Nurs Res 1989;38(3):172-7.

20. Aiken LH. Superior outcomes for magnet hospitals: the evidence base. In: McClure ML, Hinshaw AS, eds. Magnet hospitals revisited. Washington, DC: American Nurses Publishing; 2002. p. 61-81.

21. Aiken LH, Patrician PA. Measuring organizational traits of hospitals: the Revised Nursing Work Index. Nurs Res 2000 May-Jun;49:146-53.

22. Hinshaw AS. Building magnetism into health organizations. In: McClure ML, Hinshaw AS, eds. Magnet hospitals revisited: attraction and retention of professional nurses. Washington, DC: American Nurses Publishing; 2002. p. 83-102.

23. Scott JG, Sochalski J, Aiken L. Review of magnet hospital research: findings and implications for professional nursing practice. J Nurs Adm 1999 Jan; 29:9-19.

24. Abbott A. The system of professions: an essay on the division of expert labor. Chicago, IL: The University of Chicago Press; 1988.

Magnet Recognition Program Impacts

25. Lake ET. Development of the practice environment scale of the Nursing Work Index. Res Nurs Health 2002 Jun; 25:176-88.

26. Estabrooks CA, Tourangeau AE, Humphrey CK, et al. Measuring the hospital practice environment: a Canadian context. Res Nurs Health 2002 Aug; 25:256-68.

27. Choi J, Bakken S, Larson E, et al. Perceived nursing work environment of critical care nurses. Nurs Res 2004 Nov-Dec;53:370-8.

28. Aiken LH, Smith HL, Lake ET. Lower Medicare mortality among a set of hospitals known for good nursing care. Med Care 1994 Aug; 32:771-87.

29. Aiken LH, Sloane DM. Effects of organizational innovations in AIDS care on burnout among urban hospital nurses. Work Occup 1997; 24:453-77.

30. Aiken LH, Sloane DM. Effects of specialization and client differentiation on the status of nurses: the case of AIDS. J Health Soc Behav 1997;38:203-22.

31. Aiken LH, Sochalski J, Lake ET. Studying outcomes of organizational change in health services. Med Care 1997; 35(suppl):NS6-N18.

32. Aiken LH, Sloane DM, Lake ET. Satisfaction with inpatient AIDS care: a national comparison of dedicated and scattered-bed units. Med Care 1997;35:948-62.

33. Aiken LH, Lake ET, Sochalski J, et al. Design of an outcomes study of the organization of hospital AIDS care. Res Sociol Health Care 1997;14:3-26.

34. Aiken LH, Sloane DM, Klocinski JL. Hospital nurses' occupational exposure to blood: prospective, retrospective, and institutional reports. Am J Public Health 1997;87(1):103-107.

35. Aiken LH, Sloane DM, Lake ET, et al. Organization and outcomes of inpatient AIDS care. Med Care 1999;37:760-72.

36. Havens, DS. Comparing nursing infrastructure and outcomes: ANCC Magnet and nonmagnet CNE's report. Nurs Econ, 2001;19:258-66.

37. Thomas-Hawkins C, Denno M, Currier H, et al. Staff nurses' perceptions of the work environment in freestanding hemodialysis facilities. Nephrol Nurs J 2003 Aug: 30(4):377-86. [Previously published Apr:30(2):169-78.]

38. Smith H, Tallman R, Kelly K. Magnet hospital characteristics and northern Canadian nurses' job satisfaction. Can J Nurs Leadersh 2006 Sep;19(3):73-86.

39. Rondeau KV, Wagar TH. Nurse and resident satisfaction in magnet long-term care organizations: do high involvement approaches matter? J Nurs Manag 2006 Apr; 14:244-50.

40. Laschinger HK, Shamian J, Thomson D. Impact of Magnet hospital characteristics on nurses' perceptions of trust, burnout, quality of care, and work satisfaction. Nurs Econ 2001:19:209-19.

41. Laschinger HK, Almost J, Tuer-Hodes D. Workplace empowerment and magnet hospital characteristics: making the link. J Nurs Adm 2003 Jul-Aug; 33(7-8):410-22.

42. Tigert JA, Laschinger HK. Critical care nurses' perceptions of workplace empowerment, magnet hospital traits and mental health. Dynamics 2004 Winter;15(4):19-23.

43. Armstrong KJ, Laschinger H. Structural empowerment, Magnet hospital characteristics, and patient safety culture: making the link. J Nurs Care Qual 2006 Apr-Jun; 21(2):124-32.

44. Laschinger HK, Leiter MP. The impact of nursing work environments on patient safety outcomes: the mediating role of burnout/engagement. J Nurs Adm. 2006 May;36:259-67.

45. Lundstrom T, Pugliese G, Bartley J, et al. Organizational and environmental factors that affect worker health and safety and patient outcomes. Am J Infect Control 2002 Apr; 30(2):93-106.

46. Friese CR. Nurse practice environments and outcomes: implications for oncology nursing. Oncol Nurs Forum 2005 Jul 1: 32:765-72.

47. Cummings GG, Hayduk L, Estabrooks CA. Is the Nursing Work Index measuring up? Moving beyond estimating reliability to testing validity. Nurs Res 2006 Mar-Apr; 55(2):82-93.

48. Kramer M, Schmalenberg C. Magnet hospitals talk about the impact of DRGs on nursing care—Part I. Nurs Manage 1987 Sep;18(9):38-42.

49. Kramer M, Schmalenberg C. Magnet hospitals talk about the impact of DRGs on nursing care—Part II. Nurs Manage 1987 Oct: 18(10):33-6, 38-40.

50. Kramer M, Schmalenberg C. Magnet hospitals: Part I. Institutions of excellence. J Nurs Adm 1988 Jan;18(1):13-24.

Patient Safety and Quality: An Evidence-Based Handbook for Nurses

51. Kramer M, Schmalenberg C. Magnet hospitals: Part II. Institutions of excellence. J Nurs Adm 1988 Feb;18(2):11-9.

52. Kramer M, Schmalenberg C, Hafner LP. What causes job satisfaction and productivity of quality nursing care? In: Moore TF, Simendinger EA, eds. Managing the nursing shortage: a guide to recruitment and retention. Rockville, MD: Aspen; 1989. p. 12-32.

53. Peters TJ, Waterman RH. In search of excellence. New York: Harper Row Publishers; 1982.

54. Kramer M, Schmalenberg C. Job satisfaction and retention. Insights for the '90s. Part 1. Nursing 1991 Mar; 21(3):50-5.

55. Kramer M, Schmalenberg C. Job satisfaction and retention. Insights for the '90s. Part 2. Nursing 1991 Apr; 21(4):51-5.

56. Aiken LH, Havens DS, Sloane DM. The Magnet nursing services recognition program. Am J Nurs 2000 Mar;100(3):26-35; quiz 35-6.

57. Upenieks VV. The interrelationship of organizational characteristics of magnet hospitals, nursing leadership, and nursing job satisfaction. Health Care Manag (Frederick) 2003 Apr-Jun;22(2):83-98.

58. Upenieks VV. Assessing differences in job satisfaction of nurses in magnet and nonmagnet hospitals. J Nurs Adm 2002 Nov; 32:564-76.

59. Brady-Schwartz DC. Further evidence on the Magnet Recognition program: implications for nursing leaders. J Nurs Adm 2005 Sep; 35:397-403.

Magnet Recognition Program Impacts

Evidence Table 1.‡ Studies With Reputational Magnet Hospitals

Source	Environment Issue/Attribute Related to Clinical Practice	Design Type	Study Design & Study Outcome Measure(s)	Study Setting & Study Population	Key Finding(s)
Kramer and Hafner 1989[19] Kramer and Schmalenberg 1987[48-51] Kramer, Schmalenberg, and Hafner 1988[52]	Nursing Work Index (NWI), 65 items designed to measure work values representing the findings from the 1983 original magnet study Other measures: • culture of excellence, 8 items suggested by Peters and Waterman[53] • locus of control • autonomy-patient advocacy • self-concept/self-esteem • role behavior scales	Cross-sectional studies	Cross-sectional survey, interviews, observations, document review Outcomes: from NWI: • job satisfaction • perceived productivity of quality patient care	1985–86 data collection 16 reputational magnets proportionate by region, 8 comparison county, community, and medical center hospitals in Virginia Survey n = 2,236 staff nurses, 1,634 in reputational magnet and 702 in comparison group; interview n = 800+ staff nurses, 632 nurse managers/executives	Staff nurses in magnet hospitals had significantly higher scores on • job satisfaction • perceived productivity of quality care Causal model testing to predict outcomes with 31 variables produced no findings.
Kramer and Schmalenberg 1991[54, 55]	Magnet factors: • perceived adequacy of staffing • image of nurses • how nursing is valued (how important, how active, how powerful) Other measures: • culture of excellence, 39 items to represent 7 attributes	Cross-sectional studies	Cross-sectional survey Outcome: Overall job satisfaction: • organizational structure (7 items) • professional practice (5 items) • management style (5 items) • quality of leadership (4 items) • professional development (3 items)	1989–90 data collection Survey n = 939 nurses in 14 reputational magnets (from 1985–86 sample), 808 nurses in comparison "panel" sampled from 5,000 Nursing89 subscribers	Nurses in magnet hospitals had significantly more positive scores on • job satisfaction Nurses in magnet hospitals reported higher levels for • a culture of excellence • perceived adequacy of staffing • image of nursing • value of nursing

‡ To illustrate how this research has developed and expanded over time, the evidence tables in this chapter are arranged in chronological order by the data collection date for each study, when available, or publication date.

Patient Safety and Quality: An Evidence-Based Handbook for Nurses

Source	Environment Issue/Attribute Related to Clinical Practice	Design Type	Study Design & Study Outcome Measure(s)	Study Setting & Study Population	Key Finding(s)
Aiken, Smith, and Lake 1994[28]	Status as a reputational magnet hospital	Cross-sectional studies	Cross-sectional; multivariate matched sampling procedure to control for relevant hospital characteristics (e.g., teaching status, technology availability, board certification of physicians, emergency room presence), adjusting for differences in predicted mortality for Medicare patients Outcome: Medicare mortality rate (within 30 days of admission)	1988 Medicare data 39 reputational magnet hospitals (census of all available or eligible), 195 control hospitals (5 matches for each magnet) from all nonmagnet U.S. hospitals with >100 Medicare discharges	Magnet hospitals had a 4.5% lower mortality rate (95% CI (confidence interval) = 0.9 to 9.4 fewer deaths per 1,000 discharges).
Aiken and Sloane 1997[29, 30] Aiken, Sochalski, and Lake 1997[31] Aiken, Sloane and Lake 1997[32] Aiken, Lake, Sochalski 1997[33] Aiken, Sloane, and Klocinski 1997[34] Aiken, Sloane, Lake 1999[35]	Nursing Work Index–Revised (NWI-R), 57 items, with subscales for • nurse autonomy (5 items) • control over nursing practice setting (7 items) • nurse relations with physicians (2 items) • organizational support (10 items from previous 3 subscales)	Cross-sectional studies	Cross-sectional survey, needlestick reports for a 30-day period, patient interviews, patient chart abstraction Outcomes— Nurse— • job burnout • safety (needlesticks) Patient— • satisfaction with care (multi-item scale and a single-item overall rating) • mortality 30 days from admission	1991 data collection 40 medical units, 2 in each of 20 urban hospitals located throughout U.S., 10 hospitals with dedicated AIDS units, 10 matched comparable hospitals without AIDS units (scattered-bed), 2 comparison hospitals were reputational magnets, 1 more was considered magnet based on researcher knowledge of facility Survey n = 820 RNs from all employed on units ≥16 hours per week (86% response rate); interview n = 594 patients; chart outcomes for 1,205 AIDS patients	Patients with AIDS in magnet scattered-bed units had lower odds of dying than in any other setting; higher nurse-to-patient ratios were determined to be the major explanatory factor. Patient satisfaction was highest in magnet hospitals; control over nursing practice setting was determined to be the single most important explanatory factor. Nurses in magnet hospitals sustained significantly fewer needlestick injuries. Nurses in magnet hospitals and dedicated AIDS units had significantly more positive scores for emotional exhaustion, autonomy, nurse control over resources, and nurse-physician relations.

Magnet Recognition Program Impacts

Source	Environment Issue/Attribute Related to Clinical Practice	Design Type	Study Design & Study Outcome Measure(s)	Study Setting & Study Population	Key Finding(s)
Scott, Sochalski, and Aiken 1999[23]		Literature review, narrative	Search method unstated.		Summarizes findings cited in this table and synthesizes insights from these and additional magnet studies to illuminate the leadership characteristics and professional practice attributes found within reputational magnet hospitals.

Patient Safety and Quality: An Evidence-Based Handbook for Nurses

Evidence Table 2. Studies Comparing Health Care Organizations With and Without ANCC Magnet Recognition

Source	Environment Issue/Attribute Related to Clinical Practice	Design Type	Study Design & Study Outcome Measure(s)	Study Setting & Study Population	Key Finding(s)
Aiken, Havens, and Sloane 2000[56] Friese 2005[46]	NWI-R single items and subscales, Aiken et al.: • nurses' autonomy • nurses' control over the practice setting • nurse relations with physicians Practice Environment Scale/Nursing Work Index (PES/NWI), Friese: • nurse participation in hospital affairs (9 items) • nursing foundations for quality of care (10 items) • nurse manager ability, leadership, and support of nurses (5 items) • staffing and resource adequacy (4 items) • collegial nurse-physician relations (3 items) Other measures: • job characteristics (hours worked, workload, supervisory responsibilities, nonnursing duties)	Cross-sectional studies	Cross-sectional, comparative multisite observational Outcomes: • perceived quality of care • job satisfaction • intent to leave • burnout (Maslach Burnout Inventory)	1998 data collection 7 ANCC Magnets (census as of study date), 13 reputational magnets (12 from Kramer et al.'s 1985–86 sample) with 2 additional teaching hospitals included in Friese's secondary analysis Aiken et al. survey n = 2,045 RNs in medical or surgical units, 1,064 in ANCC Magnet and 981 in reputational magnet group Friese analysis n = 1,956 of which 305 = oncology nurses (155 in ANCC Magnet and 150 in comparison group) and 1,651 = nononcology nurses (755 in ANCC Magnet and 896 in comparison group)	Nurses in ANCC Magnets were significantly more likely to report • higher ratings of care quality • higher job satisfaction • less frequently feeling burned out, emotionally drained, and frustrated by their job Oncology nurses in ANCC Magnets reported nearly half the exhaustion levels of oncology nurses in the 13 reputational magnets and 2 teaching hospitals. In both analyses, most NWI-related subscale scores were significantly higher for nurses in the ANCC Magnet group; exceptions were that scores for nurse-physician relations and nurse manager ability, leadership, and support differed significantly, favoring ANCC Magnets only for oncology nurses.
Havens 2001[38]	NWI-R subscale: • organizational support Other measures: • degree restructuring implemented, 9 items	Cross-sectional studies	Cross-sectional survey; comparative Outcomes: • difficulty recruiting staff RNs (1 item) • quality of patient care (global ratings and reports of complaints)	1999–2000 data collection 21 ANCC Magnets, 35 reputational magnet hospitals (census samples of both groups) Survey n = 43 chief nurse executives, 19 in ANCC Magnet and 24 in reputational magnet group	Chief nurse executives in the ANCC Magnet group reported less difficulty recruiting RNs and were significantly more likely to report • high quality patient care • fewer patient/family complaints • organizational support for autonomy, control over practice, and nurse-physician collaboration

Magnet Recognition Program Impacts

Source	Environment Issue/Attribute Related to Clinical Practice	Design Type	Study Design & Study Outcome Measure(s)	Study Setting & Study Population	Key Finding(s)
Upenieks 2002, 2003[57,58]	Power and empowerment – Conditions of Work Effectiveness Questionnaire-II (CWEQ-II) 20 items: • 2 global items • 4 subscales to measure perceived access to opportunity, information, support, and resources	Cross-sectional studies	Cross-sectional survey Outcome: Job satisfaction - NWI-R subscales: • autonomy • nurse control over practice setting • relations between nurses and physicians Plus 3 researcher-designed subscales: • self-governance (7 items) • organizational structure (6 items) • education opportunities (6 items)	Convenience sample of 2 ANCC Magnets, 2 comparable comparison hospitals Survey n = 305 medical-surgical nurses	Nurses in the ANCC Magnet group had significantly higher scores on • job satisfaction • power and empowerment
Brady-Schwartz 2005[59]	Status as ANCC-recognized Magnet	Cross-sectional studies	Cross-sectional survey; quantitative, descriptive correlational Outcome: • overall job satisfaction (total McCloskey Mueller Satisfaction Scale score; subscales: extrinsic rewards, scheduling, family/work balance, coworkers, interaction, professional opportunities, praise and recognition, control/responsibility) • intention to leave (Anticipated Turnover Scale)	3 ANCC Magnets, 3 comparison hospitals Survey n = 470 RNs, 173 in ANCC Magnet and 297 in comparison group	Nurses in ANCC Magnet group had significantly higher overall job satisfaction, including significant subscale differences for professional opportunities, control/responsibility, and extrinsic rewards. Higher overall job satisfaction correlated with stronger perceptions of voluntarily remaining in current position.

Patient Safety and Quality: An Evidence-Based Handbook for Nurses

Evidence Table 3. Studies of Magnet Characteristics

Source	Environment Issue/Attribute Related to Clinical Practice	Design Type	Study Design & Study Outcome Measure(s)	Study Setting & Study Population	Key Finding(s)
Laschinger, Shamian, and Thomson 2001[40]	Magnet characteristics—NWI-R subscales: • nurse autonomy • nurse control over practice setting • nurses' relations with physicians Other measures: • trust and confidence in management — Interpersonal Trust at Work Scale • burnout—The Human Services Survey, 3 components (emotional exhaustion, depersonalization, decreased personal accomplishments)	Cross-sectional studies	Cross-sectional survey Outcomes: • job satisfaction • perceived quality of care • perceived quality of unit	Ontario, Canada Survey n = 3,016 staff nurses from medical-surgical settings (subsample from a stratified random sample) in 135 hospitals	Model testing with these variables explained 39–40% of the variance with either job satisfaction or nurse-assessed quality as the outcome. Magnet characteristics influenced job satisfaction and perceptions of care quality with trust in management and emotional exhaustion as important mediators. Higher levels of magnet characteristics were associated with higher levels of trust in management and lower levels of burnout.
Thomas-Hawkins, Denno, Currier 2003[37]	Magnet characteristics – PES/NWI subscales (some items adapted to reflect setting): • nurse participation in hospital affairs • nursing foundations for quality of care • nurse manager ability, leadership, and support of nurses • staffing and resource adequacy • collegial nurse-physician relations	Cross-sectional studies	Cross-sectional survey Outcome: intentions to leave job in next year (1 item)	United States 1,000 staff nurses working in freestanding hemodialysis facilities (random sample from American Nephrology Nurses' Association members)	Nurses who intended to leave their jobs reported significantly lower levels of magnet characteristics represented by all of the PES/NWI subscales except for collegial relations between nurses and physicians.

Magnet Recognition Program Impacts

Source	Environment Issue/Attribute Related to Clinical Practice	Design Type	Study Design & Study Outcome Measure(s)	Study Setting & Study Population	Key Finding(s)
Laschinger, Almost, and Tuer-Hodes 2003[41]	Magnet characteristics—NWI-R subscales: • nurse autonomy • nurse control over practice setting • nurses' relations with physicians Other measures: Empowerment • CWEQ-II, 4 subscales: access to opportunity, information, support, and resources Job Activities Scale-II, 3 items: perceptions of formal power • Organizational Relationships Scale-II, 4 items: perceptions of informal power	Cross-sectional studies	Cross-sectional survey data from 3 independent studies; predictive, nonexperimental Outcomes: • Global Job Satisfaction Questionnaire (Studies 1, 3) • Nurse Job Satisfaction Questionnaire (Study 2)	Ontario, Canada Study 1: survey n = 233 randomly selected staff nurses from urban tertiary care hospitals throughout Ontario Study 2: survey n = 263 randomly selected staff nurses from 3 rural community hospitals in a western Ontario network of 8 Study 3: survey n = 55 acute care nurse practitioners from urban tertiary care hospitals throughout Ontario	For staff nurses, empowerment and magnet characteristics were significant independent predictors of job satisfaction; for nurse practitioners, the combination of empowerment and magnet characteristics significantly predicted job satisfaction. Average ratings on empowerment and magnet characteristics were moderate for staff nurses and higher for nurse practitioners. Total scores on empowerment and magnet characteristics were strongly correlated for all three samples; the most strongly related empowerment features were access to resources for staff nurses and access to information for nurse practitioners. All empowerment dimensions related significantly to perceptions of autonomy; access to resources related most strongly to control over practice environment; and informal power related most strongly to nurse-physician relationships.

Patient Safety and Quality: An Evidence-Based Handbook for Nurses

Source	Environment Issue/Attribute Related to Clinical Practice	Design Type	Study Design & Study Outcome Measure(s)	Study Setting & Study Population	Key Finding(s)
Tigert and Laschinger 2004[42]	Magnet characteristics – NWI-R subscales: • nurse autonomy • nurse control over practice setting • nurses' relations with physicians Other measures: Empowerment • CWEQ-II, 4 subscales: access to opportunity, information, support, and resources • Job Activities Scale-II, 3 items: perceptions of formal power • Organizational Relationships Scale-II, 4 items: perceptions of informal power	Cross-sectional studies	Cross-sectional, correlational survey design Outcomes: mental health • State of Mind subscale (5 items) from the Pressure Management Indicator • Emotional Exhaustion subscale (6 items) from the Maslach Burnout Inventory	Ontario, Canada; Data collected 2001 Survey n = 75 critical care nurses, a subsample of 239 nurses working in teaching hospitals (randomly selected from College of Nurses of Ontario)	The combined effects of empowerment and magnet characteristics explained 19% of the variance in burnout and 12% of the variance in state of mind. Empowerment related significantly and positively to perceptions of magnet characteristics; however, only empowerment was a significant independent predictor of emotional exhaustion, and only magnet characteristics were a significant predictor of state of mind.
Rondeau and Wagar 2006[39]	Magnet similarity represented by employer-of-choice strength (7 items, e.g., how establishment views, values, treats its nursing personnel; how staff and community view its treatment of nurses) Other magnet characteristics measures: • high involvement (high commitment) work practices (10 items) • progressive, participatory decisionmaking workplace culture (3 items) • training support (10 items)	Cross-sectional studies	Cross-sectional survey Outcomes: • resident satisfaction (3 items) • nurse turnover and vacancy rates • nurse satisfaction (3 items)	Canada Data collected 2003 Survey n = 114 nurse executives sampled from all long-term care organizations (nursing homes) in western Canada with ≥35 beds	Higher scores on magnet employer-of-choice strength were significantly associated with • higher resident satisfaction • lower turnover and vacancy rates • higher nurse satisfaction • high involvement work practices • progressive decisionmaking practices • nurse training opportunities and assistance

Magnet Recognition Program Impacts

Source	Environment Issue/Attribute Related to Clinical Practice	Design Type	Study Design & Study Outcome Measure(s)	Study Setting & Study Population	Key Finding(s)
Smith, Tallman, and Kelly 2006[38]	Magnet characteristics categories: • supportive management (5 items) • professional autonomy and responsibility (4 items) • nurse-physician working relationship (2 items) • nurse-manager working relationship (2 items)	Cross-sectional studies	Cross-sectional survey, interviews Outcome: job satisfaction (3 items from Job Diagnostic Survey)	Canada Survey n = 123 nurses in diverse clinical areas from 13 rural northwestern hospitals recruited via circulating letter/flyer	All magnet characteristics items were significantly but modestly correlated with job satisfaction except for the 2 items measuring nurse-physician relationship and 1 of the 4 autonomy items.
Armstrong and Laschinger 2006[43]	Magnet characteristics – PES-NWI subscales: • nurse participation in hospital affairs • nursing foundations for quality of care • nurse manager ability, leadership, and support of nurses • staffing and resource adequacy • collegial nurse-physician relations Other measures: Structural empowerment – CWEQ-II, 2 global items and 6 components: access to opportunity, information, support, resources, formal power, and informal power	Cross-sectional studies	Cross-sectional survey; exploratory; predictive, nonexperimental Outcome measure: Safety Climate Survey	Canada 40 staff nurses working in a small community hospital in central Canada	The combination of structural empowerment and magnet characteristics was a significant predictor of perceptions of patient safety climate. Overall empowerment significantly positively related to all magnet characteristics, with total empowerment most strongly related to use of a nursing model of care and good nursing leadership on the unit.

Patient Safety and Quality: An Evidence-Based Handbook for Nurses

Source	Environment Issue/Attribute Related to Clinical Practice	Design Type	Study Design & Study Outcome Measure(s)	Study Setting & Study Population	Key Finding(s)
Laschinger and Leiter 2006[44]	Magnet characteristics – PES-NWI subscales: • nurse participation in hospital affairs • nursing foundations for quality of care • nurse manager ability, leadership, and support of nurses • staffing and resource adequacy • collegial nurse-physician relations Other measures: Maslach Burnout Inventory–Human Service Scale, 3 subscales: • emotional exhaustion (9 items) • depersonalization (5 items) • personal accomplishment (8 items)	Cross-sectional studies	Cross-sectional survey Outcome measure: adverse events (nurse-reported frequency of occurrence of negative patient events in past year: • falls • nosocomial infections • medication errors • patient complaints)	Canada Survey n = 8,597 nurses (4,606 from a stratified random sample of licensing registry lists in Ontario and 3,991 from a census sample of acute care nurses in Alberta), a subset of participants in the *International Survey of Hospital Staffing and Organization of Patient Outcomes* conducted in 5 countries	With all measured components included in the model, structural equation modeling analysis showed direct and indirect effects of all environment factors on patient safety outcomes partially mediated by burnout. Both staffing adequacy and use of a nursing model of care directly affected patient safety outcomes. Staffing adequacy directly affected emotional exhaustion, and use of a nursing care model directly affected personal accomplishment. Nursing leadership played a fundamental role in relation to policy involvement, staffing adequacy, RN-MD relationships, and support for a nursing (vs. medical) model of care.

The Business Case for Magnet®

Karen Drenkard, PhD, RN, NEA-BC, FAAN

Adapted and reprinted with permission from *Journal of Nursing Administration*,
Vol. 40, No. 6, pp. 263–271
© 2010 Wolters Kluwer Health & Wilkins/Lippincott Williams & Wilkins

A culture of discipline is not a principle of business; it is a principle of greatness.
Jim Collins

In life and business, there are two cardinal sins. The first is to act precipitously without thought and the second is to not act at all.
Carl Icahn

This chapter describes the role of the chief nurse executive (CNE) in delivering a business case for the Journey to Magnet Excellence™. Calculating a return on investment provides clear measurement of benefits of the credential and can be used to evaluate upfront resources that result in a longer-term gain. The range of cost savings that can possibly be achieved for a typical 500-bed hospital is presented. Although not every hospital will achieve the level of performance implied by the national assumptions, securing only a modicum of the potential level of cost improvement will assure a multifold return on the investment required.

One of the important responsibilities of a CNE is to share information with the rest of the executive team about programs and efforts that are beneficial to the delivery of patient care. This includes securing the support of the Chief Executive Officer and others on the executive level. When a financial investment is required, stating a strong and convincing case is a key strategy for engaging the executive decision-makers, including the chief financial officer. In the case of a decision to pursue Magnet® status, the support of the entire executive team is a necessity. In 2008, a new Magnet Model was developed based on scholarly review and statistical analysis (Wolf et al., 2008).

Figure 11-1. The Magnet Model

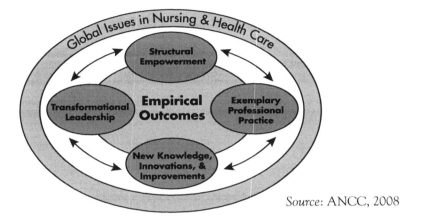

Source: ANCC, 2008

The new Magnet Model offers a framework for organizing a nursing services division (Figure 11-1). Magnet status is not a prize or an award; it is a credential of organizational recognition of nursing excellence. The process requires organizations to develop, disseminate, and enculturate evidence-based criteria that result in a positive work environment for nurses and, by extension, all employees. It is a multiyear commitment, and requires the full support of the leadership team, the hospital healthcare organization's administration, and the board of directors.

HISTORY OF THE MAGNET RECOGNITION PROGRAM

During the nursing shortage of the 1980s a group of insightful nurse researchers took a unique approach to understanding the shortage of that decade. They led a nationwide research study, commissioned by the American Academy of Nursing, that investigated what was right with the hospital workplaces that had low RN vacancy and turnover rates. This groundbreaking research was described in 1983 in *Magnet Hospitals: Attraction and Retention of Professional Nurses* (McClure et al., 1983), and identified themes that were later called the Forces of Magnetism. This research base served as the foundation of the creation of the Magnet Recognition Program®, a program of the American Nurses Credentialing Center. To date (2010), over 377 domestic and international hospitals and healthcare organizations have met the Sources of Evidence for nursing excellence and are recognized as Magnet hospitals.

WHY CONSIDER MAGNET AS A FRAMEWORK FOR NURSING SERVICES?

The Magnet Recognition Program is used by many CNEs as a roadmap for excellence in nursing services, and can serve as a framework for organizing a hospital nursing delivery system. This chapter articulates the steps for development of a business case for Magnet recognition in order to obtain organizational support. The chapter also presents the research and financial evidence to build and present the case for embarking on the Magnet journey.

WHAT IS A BUSINESS CASE?

The business case is a proposal that can assist an organization or executive in presenting the reasoning for beginning a change project or group of tasks. The evaluative nature of a business case assists in the decision "to go or not to go" with a specific initiative, as well as evaluation of one decision or project against others. In the case of seeking Magnet recognition, the CNE can present organizational change, business, and financial implications and benefits in a formal presentation that all members of the executive team can understand. This helps to begin the process of acquiring support, and serves as a milestone in the Magnet process for approval and sponsorship of the executive team and the board of directors.

Weaver and Sorrells-Jones (2007) describe the business case as a strategic tool for change and encourage the development of the business case as a key tactic in determining choices among multiple options, especially in tough economic times. They describe five key information areas that need to be covered in the business plan, including degree of strategic fit, program objectives, review of options, affordability, and achievability (Weaver & Sorrells-Jones, 2007, p. 415). Measurements for addressing key milestones as a way to measure progress should be developed and included. In addition, the business case should answer the question, "How will this effort solve the issues we face?"

The business case includes the reason for the project, the expected business results and benefits, and the costs and the risks. The case serves as a way to capture knowledge, functions as a basis for receiving funding and approval, helps prioritize the project against other competing initiatives that might also require funding, and secures a consistent message to all key stakeholders in the process (Prosci, 2009, 2010). Formal business cases can ensure that the investment has value and importance, that the project will be properly managed, that there is capability to deliver, that the program or project is adequately resourced, and that the project has the long-term support required for success (Value Delivery Management, 2009).

BUILDING THE BUSINESS CASE FOR MAGNET

The business case should include the purpose statement and the value added of embarking on the initiative. In this case, why would your hospital commit to the Journey to Magnet Excellence? Linking the purpose of the initiative to the mission of the organization is an effective way to align the decision to pursue Magnet with the needs of the patients and community. Within the framework of the organization's strategic plan and the nursing services' strategic plan, determining the degree of fit is critical. The CNE needs to strategically align the priorities of the organization with the framework for nursing excellence. Viewing nursing's contribution to the organization as a strategic differentiator of high-quality care is one perspective that the Magnet journey fully supports.

With nursing as the primary service that is provided in hospitals, recognition that your hospital's nursing services are in the top 5%–10% of the nation's hospitals is a mark of excellence that has a strong value proposition for key stakeholders, including physicians and consumers. A growing body of research indicates that Magnet hospitals have higher percentages of satisfied RNs, lower RN turnover and vacancies, improved clinical outcomes, excellent nurse autonomy and decision-making capabilities, and improved patient satisfaction (Aiken et al., 1997; Aiken et al., 2000; Aiken et al., 2008; Armstrong & Laschinger, 2006; Armstrong et al., 2008; Brady-Schwartz, 2005; Havens & Aiken, 1999; Kramer, 1990; Lacey et al., 2007; Laschinger et al., 2003; Scott et al., 1999; Tigert & Laschinger, 2004; Ulrich et al., 2007).

Table 11-1. Return-on-Investment Opportunities: The Evidence

Human Resources
- Increased RN retention and lower nurse burnout (Aiken et al., 1997; Jones & Gates, 2007; Lacey et al., 2007)
- Decreased RN vacancy rate and RN turnover rate (Jones & Gates, 2007; McConnell, 1999; Upenieks, 2003)

Costs
- Reduction in RN agency rates (Upenieks, 2003)
- Reduction in staff needle-stick rates (Clarke et al., 2002; Jagger et al., 1990; Neisner & Raymond, 2002)
- Reduction in staff musculoskeletal and other injuries (Stone & Gershon, 2006)
- Marketing Return on Investment – publication in lieu of ads (Woods, 2002a, 2002b; Woods & Cardin, 2002)

Service
- Increased patient satisfaction (Gardner et al., 2007)
- Increased RN satisfaction (Brady-Schwartz, 2005; Cimmiotti et al., 2005; Laschinger et al., 2004; Smith et al., 2006; Waldman et al., 2004)

Quality and Safety
- Decreased mortality rates (Aiken et al., 1994; Aiken et al., 1997; Aiken et al., 1999)
- Decreased pressure ulcers (Berquist-Beringer et al., 2009; Goode & Blegen, 2009; Rosenberg, 2009)
- Decreased falls (Bates et al., 1995; Dunton et al., 2004; Dunton et al., 2007; Hitcho et al., 2004; Hook & Winchel, 2006; Nurmi & Luthje, 2002)
- Patient Safety and improved quality (Armstrong & Laschinger, 2006; Armstrong et al., 2008; Hines & Yu, 2009; Hughes et al., 2009; Laschinger & Leiter, 2006; Stone et al., 2007)

Table 11-1 presents evidence related to return on investment opportunities. It displays some literature-based measures of quality, service, cost, and human resources that are worth evaluating in organizations to determine if the Journey to Magnet Excellence could be a strategic driver toward improvement. Although costs and return on investment are important, they are not the only reason for deciding to pursue Magnet recognition. Often having the multi-layer framework for quality improvement efforts and a mechanism for engaging staff in decision-making is a helpful tool for a new CNE or for CNEs looking for a way to energize and motivate their teams. Team building, collaborating across disciplines, and building staff engagement are harder to quantify, but are often results of the Magnet journey.

When building the business case, it is important to identify critical factors that will maximize success in reaching the end goal of obtaining Magnet status. A Magnet gap analysis is a helpful first step and should be completed before the business case is presented to the board. With the gap analysis, the CNE is in a better position to completely identify what resources and support will be needed to meet the Magnet program Sources of Evidence. In addition, the gap analysis will guide the timeline for completion of any areas that need strengthening. Critical success factors also inform a discussion of strategic risks that need to be shared with the executive team.

What, if any, are the downsides of pursuing Magnet status? How can the risk of failure be minimized? These will be different for each organization, but include the willingness of the organization to engage in the Magnet journey as a peer-reviewed credentialing process with some degree of risk in the event that not all of the criteria are met. The achievement of Magnet status is a high bar, and the support of the entire executive team and the board is necessary (Doloresco, 2004; Poduska, 2005). The executive leadership has a responsibility to ensure that Magnet status can be sustained over time. The business case should also include a high-level timeline, assigned accountability for the executive ownership of the work plan, and an implementation, communication, and evaluation plan for monitoring the progress toward achieving Magnet recognition.

THE LITERATURE BASE OF EVIDENCE FOR QUALITY, SERVICE, AND COST

One good way to build the case for pursuing Magnet designation is to provide the evidence base to the executive leadership. This selected review of the literature pertaining to Magnet status benefits gives CNEs an array of choices that can be linked to the needs of their organization. In addition, opportunities for cost savings can be identified by understanding the basis for improvement opportunities.

Quality

Increasingly, nursing is being recognized as a major contributor to quality and safety in patient care (Armstrong & Laschinger, 2006; Hughes et al., 2009; Laschinger & Leiter, 2006; Stone et al., 2007). Decreased pressure ulcers and decreased falls have been linked to Magnet hospitals (Aiken et al., 1999; Berquist-Beringer et al., 2009; Goode & Blegen, 2009). Results of a cross-sectional design of hospitalized patients with hip fractures led to conclusions that, including Medicare beneficiaries, those who had received care for a hip fracture were less likely to develop a decubitus ulcer in a Magnet hospital (Rosenberg, 2009). Other studies support the advantages of Magnet hospitals compared to non-Magnet hospitals related to skin integrity, and cost savings opportunities of $43,180 per case (Beckrich & Aronovitch, 1999; Goode & Blegen, 2009; Hines & Yu, 2009).

Another nurse-sensitive indicator that has been demonstrated as having lower rates in Magnet hospitals is patient falls. Multiple studies report fall rates in Magnet hospitals 10% lower than in non-Magnet hospitals (Dunton et al., 2007). Compared with the reported rates in general (Bates et al., 1995; Dunton et al., 2004; Hitcho et al., 2004; Hook & Winchel, 2006; Shorr et al., 2008) of 3 to 4 per 1000 patient-days, savings can be determined based on the reduced frequency of patient falls in Magnet hospitals.

Patient Safety

Recent studies have evaluated the linkages between the work environment for nurses and the patient safety climate (Armstrong & Laschinger, 2006; Armstrong et al., 2008; Hughes & Chang, 2009; Laschinger & Leiter, 2006; Stone et al., 2007). In these studies, overall magnet hospital characteristics were significantly and positively related to a patient safety climate in the work setting. The combined effect of increased access to empowerment structures and Magnet hospital characteristics was significantly related to higher perceived safety climate.

Decreased Mortality

The two compelling studies from the original Magnet research were conducted by nurse scientist Dr. Linda Aiken. For the Medicare mortality study (Aiken, Clarke, & Cheung et al., 2003; Aiken et al., 2000; Aiken, Lake, & Sochalski et al., 1997; Aiken & Sloane, 1997a, 1997b; Aiken, Sloane, & Klocinski, 1997; Aiken, Sloane, & Lake, 1997; Aiken et al., 1994; Aiken, Sochalski, & Lake, 1997; Potter et al., 2003), characteristics of a Magnet environment were measured and associated with significantly better outcomes for mortality 30 days from admission. In addition, a significantly better outcome was determined for nurse safety, job burnout, and patient satisfaction.

Service

Magnet hospitals have a long history of positive nurse and work satisfaction linked to increased autonomy in practice, structural empowerment, participation in decision-making opportunities, and a positive work environment (Cimmiotti et al., 2005; Laschinger et al., 2001; Laschinger et al., 2007; Rondeau & Wagar, 2006; Schmalenberg & Kramer, 2008; Smith et al., 2006). Ulrich et al. (2007) evaluated areas of work and the professional practice environment in a study of 735 RNs in Magnet and non-Magnet facilities. Their findings revealed that RNs in Magnet organizations reported higher satisfaction with their present job (85% very or somewhat satisfied) than did RNs who work in non-Magnet organizations (p<0.05).

COST OPPORTUNITIES FOR MAGNET HOSPITALS

Turnover

Early work by Kramer and Schmalenberg (1988a, 1988b; The Advisory Board Company, 2000) found that outcomes were better in two areas in Magnet hospitals. These were high nurse job satisfaction as measured by "being a good place to work" and high-quality care as measured by being a "good place to practice nursing." In addition, the ability of these hospitals to recruit and retain nurses led to lower vacancy and turnover rates.

Lacey et al. (2007) examined the difference between nurses' scores (n=3337) on organizational support, workload, satisfaction, and intent to stay among Magnet, Magnet-aspiring, and non-Magnet hospitals. Magnet hospitals had better scores than non-Magnet hospitals, with an implication that Magnet hospital nurses were more likely to be retained than nurses working in non-Magnet hospitals.

Costs and benefits of reducing nurse turnover were identified by Jones and Gates (2007) in an attempt to develop a business case for nurse retention. The Advisory Board (2000) reports turnover costs of one RN at $42,000–$64,000 depending on specialty area due to costs of orientation and lost productivity. Turnover costs have been estimated to range between 0.75 and 2.0 times the salary of the departing RN (McConnell, 1999) and generally accepted at one times the cost of an RN salary (Jones & Gates, 2007). Nurse retention benefits identified by Jones and Gates (2007) and others (Lavizzo-Mourey & Verplanck, 2009; Upenieks, 2003) include reduction in recruitment costs, reduction in orientation costs, productivity gains, decreased patient errors and improved quality of care, increased levels of trust and accountability, and deep organizational knowledge.

Vacancy Rate

Historically, during economic downturns, the vacancy rate for RNs has traditionally dropped, but soon returns to pre-recession levels once the economy returns. This is due to a "false impression that the shortage may be over, generating complacency in the industry" (American Hospital Association, 2007). The Magnet recognition Sources of Evidence and structures and processes for nursing services support a positive work environment that historically contributes to lower RN vacancy rates. The current vacancy rate at Magnet hospitals as of October 2009 was 3.64% compared to reported national vacancy averages in 2007 of 8.1%–16%, depending on the specialty and the region of the country (Magnet Recognition Program, 2009).

Agency Use

Upenieks (2003) identified a cost-benefit equation based on the costs of Magnet designation and the offsetting costs of decreased nursing turnover. The decrease in agency utilization was calculated on a sample cost–benefit ratio of several 300-bed acute-care hospitals. With an assumption of the reduction of a range of 5 to 20 agency shifts per day at $40 to $60 per hour differential costs per day, the potential for cost savings was calculated at several million dollars in a 300-bed hospital.

Occupational Health Injuries: Needle-Stick Injuries, Musculoskeletal Injuries, and Blood and Body Fluid Exposures

Multiple studies (Clarke et al., 2002; Havens & Aiken, 1999; Jagger et al., 1990) report up to a one-third reduction in needle-stick injuries in Magnet facilities at a cost of $405 per event. In testimony to the U. S. House Workforce Protections SubCommittee of the Committee on Education and Labor, Dr. Linda Rosenstock testified that a working ratio is 30 needle-stick injuries per 100 hospital beds. The Center for Disease Control reports 385,000 needle-stick injuries per year (Wilburn, 2004), which equals an average of 67.5 per hospital. Occupational health injuries for musculoskeletal injuries and blood and body fluid exposures are also lower in hospitals with Magnet status (Nelson et al., 2006; Stone & Gershon, 2006). Costs per musculoskeletal injury ranged from $50,000 to $100,000 per injury per nurse. By determining the needle-stick injury rates and musculoskeletal injuries before or while on the Magnet journey and tracking rates, a cost–benefit can be determined for the hospital based on lower rates in Magnet hospitals.

Patient Falls

There is growing evidence that Magnet hospitals have lower rates of patient falls than non-Magnet hospitals (Bates et al., 1995; Dunton et al., 2004; Dunton et al., 2007; Hitcho et al., 2004; Hook & Winchel, 2006; Nurmi & Luthje, 2002). Hines and Yu (2009) described a cost per hospitalization for patient falls of $33,894. They described the number of preventable injuries in the United States for fiscal year 2007 of 193,566 falls. Unruh (2008) estimates costs per fall at a range of $1,019 to $4,235 per case, with a rate of 3.73 falls per 1,000 patient-days. Magnet hospitals have a reported 10.3% lower fall rates.

Pressure Ulcers

Several studies have linked Magnet hospitals to decreased pressure ulcer rates (Berquist-Beringer et al., 2009; Goode & Blegen, 2009; Rosenberg, 2009). Mills also reported lower decubitus ulcer rates among adult, medical-surgical patients in Magnet versus non-Magnet hospitals in a 2008 study. Hines and Yu (2009) report that the number of cases of pressure ulcer stages 3 and 4 in the United States is at 257,412 annually. This would average 51.5 cases per hospital. Magnet hospitals have an improved rate of 5%, which would equal 2.5 fewer cases. A daily cost for medical and surgical patients was estimated at $5,177 (Dall et al., 2009).

Marketing Return on Investment

An identified benefit of having Magnet status is the marketing opportunities that come to Magnet facilities with publications, presentations, and other opportunities for exposure at the national level. This replaces the cost of advertisements that might otherwise need to be bought at market rates. In a business case analysis completed by the James A. Haley Veterans' Hospital (Doloresco, 2004), the page rate was calculated at $10,000 per advertisement.

Other Benefits

In addition to the research-based evidence, there are anecdotal and qualitative benefits to having Magnet status that may not be included in a cost–benefit analysis but do impact the overall health of an organization. Bond ratings and risk management assessments have included Magnet designation in their criteria and *U.S. News & World Report* added Magnet designation to its criteria for national best hospitals as a measure of quality and nursing excellence (Tuazon, 2007). There are reputational benefits of holding Magnet designation, too.

THE MAGNET SOURCES OF EVIDENCE

In addition to requirements that nurse satisfaction, patient satisfaction, and clinical outcome measures are above the midpoint of the benchmarking data points, there are Magnet Sources of Evidence that will capture improvements in quality and cost. There are at least three Sources of Evidence that encourage nurses to work on cost improvement. These are illustrated in Table 11-2. A review of the actual examples of Sources of Evidence submitted to the Magnet Recognition Program from June 2009 to December 2009 reveals cost savings and improvements of $5,000 to $20,000 for each nurse-driven improvement project per year.

Table 11-2. Sources of Evidence That Support Cost Improvements

1. TL3. The strategic planning structure and process used by nursing to improve the healthcare system's effectiveness and efficiency and TL3EO, the outcome that resulted from the planning in TL3.
2. EP12. How nurses analyze data to guide decisions regarding unit and department budget formulation, implementation, monitoring, and evaluation.
3. EP33EO. How the allocation or re-allocation of resources improved the quality of nursing care.

OVERALL FINANCIAL RETURN

There has been agreement in the literature that there is an overall financial return of Magnet designation (DeSilets & Pinkerton, 2005; Doloresco, 2004; Dunton et al., 2009; Hassmiller & Christopher, 2009; Havens, 2001; Jones & Gates, 2007; McConnell, 1999; Robert Wood Johnson Foundation, 2009). DeSilets and Pinkerton (2005) document the financial return on investment, including improved retention and decreased turnover, improved satisfaction, improved quality and safety, increased customer attraction for hospital selection, and superior business results with a climb in operating margin from 4% to 16% due to investment in nursing services rather than cutting expenses of salaries and staffing levels. The ability to engage the staff in business and operational review of business outcomes resulted in the staff participating greatly in improved efficiency and effectiveness at the unit levels (Havens & Johnston, 2004).

Each project that results in cost savings, cost avoidance, or increased revenue should be well documented by the CNE and monitored and evaluated during the Magnet journey (Gelinas, 2002). The value of professional nursing was quantified by Dall et al. (2009) and provided an economic value and monetary assessment of the value of nurse staffing that impacts patient care quality. Their evaluation concluded that adding RNs to the patient bedside would decrease hospital days and result in medical savings. The findings "strengthen the economic case for hospital investment in nursing" (p. 104).

DETERMINING THE RETURN ON INVESTMENT: DEVELOPING YOUR BUSINESS CASE

Calculating a return on investment provides clear measurement of benefits of a program and has been used to evaluate programs that require upfront resources that result in a longer-term gain. It is an important part of a business case and can add information to the decision-making process (Sandhusen et al., 2004). For the purposes of this exercise, a case study approach is taken. Assumptions are made based on the evidence for quality, service, and cost returns. The case assumes a "typical" 500-bed hospital and compares average Magnet hospital characteristics and outcomes to national averages.

The Investment

There are direct costs associated with the process of obtaining Magnet recognition status. For the purposes of this business case, the costs should be those that are over and above the normal costs for running a nursing care service in a hospital. These costs include Magnet application fees, appraiser fees, site visit costs, and document preparation. These direct costs range from $46,000 to $251,000 depending on bed size and resource decisions made by the organization. Each organization needs to determine what its resource needs are during the Magnet journey and determine total costs.

The Return on Investment

Table 11-3 provides assumptions of the difference between a 500-bed Magnet hospital and a 500-bed non-Magnet hospital. Table 11-4 demonstrates potential capture of financial improvements in areas of quality, service, and costs. Based on the literature of improvements in Magnet hospitals, and using the data assumptions of a typical 500-bed hospital, cost opportunities and a potential return on investment can be determined for a hospital. The range of cost savings that can be achieved for a typical 500-bed hospital is estimated between $2,308,350 and $2,323,350. Based on estimates of direct costs associated with achieving Magnet recognition, which range from $46,000 to $251,000, the potential resulting return on investment is compelling. Although not every hospital will achieve the level of performance implied by the national assumptions, securing only a modicum of this level of improvement will ensure a multifold return on the investment required.

Table 11-3. Assumptions About 500-Bed Magnet and Non-Magnet Hospitals

Assumptions	Magnet Hospitals*	Non-Magnet Hospitals
RN turnover	11.14%	15-18% (VHA, 2002)
RN vacancy	3.64%	8.1-16% (ANCC, 2010)
Total RN FTEs	1,184	1,184
Direct care provider RN FTEs	1,063	1,063
Admissions	28,905	28,905
ALOS	4.66 d	4.66 d
Net revenue	556 million	556 million
No. of needle-stick injuries annually	100 (1/3 lower than non-Magnet hospitals)	150 (Clarke et al., 2002; Havens & Aiken, 1999; Jagger, 1990)
RN tenure	9.5 years	
Licensed average beds	734	
Average daily census	490	

Abbreviations: FTEs, full-time equivalents; ALOS, average length of stay.
* Data from Magnet Recognition Program® data set.

Table 11-4. Potential Capture of Cost Improvements

Benefit Category	Assumptions About Benefit	500-Bed Hospital Potential Cost Savings
Clinical quality *Pressure ulcers*	Assume 2.5 cases improvement x $43,180 (Hines & Yu, 2009), cost/case	$107,950
Decreased falls	Cost for falls $1019–$4253 (Unruh, 2008) Magnet hospitals have 10.3% lower fall rates (if average falls assumed 38 cases/hospital then 3.8 fewer cases) 3.8 × $3,000 = $11,400	$11,400
Service *Nurse* *Satisfaction*	Higher nurse engagement contributes to improved turnover, lower vacancy rates and improved patient satisfaction	Savings captured in improved RN turnover and vacancy

Table 11-4. Potential Capture of Cost Improvements (cont.)

Benefit Category	Assumptions About Benefit	500-Bed Hospital Potential Cost Savings
Cost: *Improved RN vacancy and turnover and agency costs for 500-Bed hospital*	Assume: 1. 8.1% RN vacancy non-Magnet – 3.45% vacancy Magnet = 4.65% improvement in RN vacancy in Magnet facilities 2. 3.45% vacancy × 1063 RNs = 36.6 RNs vacant Magnet facility 3. 8.1% vacancy × 1063 RNs = 86.1 RNs vacant non-Magnet facility 4. Agency capture at premium pay differential rate = $20/hr 5. Agency hours for each FTE = 2,080 × $25 premium = $52,000/FTE 6. 1 FTE agency use saved for every 100 beds 7. 500-bed hospital = 5 FTEs agency 8. 5 FTEs × $52,000 = $250,000 agency cost capture 9. Difference of Magnet vs non-Magnet vacancies = 49.5 direct RN care providers × $42,000/yr = $2,079,000	$2,079,000
Needle-stick injuries (Clarke et al., 2002)	Cost of sero-conversion due to needle-stick = $500/stick (Clark, et al.2002) showed 1/3 reduction in RN needle-stick injuries If 500-bed hospital = 150 needle-stick injuries 1/3 Reduction target = 50 needle-stick injuries × $500 = savings from fewer needle-stick injuries	$25,000
Improvement due to Sources of Evidence in Magnet requirements for efficiency and effectiveness	Review of 2008 documentation submissions reflects cost savings range from $5,000 to $20,000 on nurse-driven improvement projects	$5,000–$20,000
Marketing return on investment —publication in lieu of advertisements (Veterans Affairs business case)	Assume 8 publications and presentations from hospital as result of RN research productivity at replacement ad cost of $10,000 per event if placed in major publication as paid advertisement (VA, 2004)	$80,000
TOTAL RANGE OF RETURN ON INVESTMENT	Depending on which savings hospital achieves, range of return on investment	$2,308,350–$2,323,350

PRESENTING THE CASE: SUMMARY

Weaver and Sorrell-Jones (2007) advocate preparing the business case to both present and persuade key leadership in the organization. This requires establishing the credibility of the CNE as a presenter, finding common ground about the goals that are being achieved by the organization, displaying compelling evidence, and connecting with the audience, in this case the executive team (p. 418).

Studies are increasingly adding to the evidence that link nursing care and nursing levels to the ability to improve patient care outcomes and decrease staff turnover (Hassmiller & Christopher, 2009). Understanding the data and being able to articulate the potential for a strong nursing service that results in decreased costs, improved productivity, and improved healthcare outcomes can influence the level of support for the process of participating in the Magnet Recognition Program. The CNE needs to develop and sharpen skills to speak directly to the business community and encourage its support for investing in nursing as a way to improve safety and quality in patient care (Hassmiller & Christopher, 2009).

The CNE's responsibilities include articulating the value of nursing services within a context of excellence in patient care, safety, quality, and the professional development of staff. Magnet recognition is a framework and a model that has proven results in reducing costs through increasing nursing satisfaction, patient satisfaction, and clinical outcomes.

REFERENCES

All URLs retrieved September 12, 2010.

Aiken, L. H., Clarke, S. P., Cheung, R. B., Sloane, D. M., & Silber, J. H. (2003). Education levels of hospital nurses and patient mortality. *Journal of the American Medical Association, 290*(12), 1–8.

Aiken, L. H., Clarke, S. P., & Sloane, D. M. et al. (2008). Effects of hospital care environment on patient mortality and nurses outcomes. *Journal of Nursing Administration, 38*(5), 223–229.

Aiken, L. H., Clarke, S. P., Sloane, D. M., Sochalski, J., & Silber, J. H. (2000). Hospital nurse staffing and patient mortality, nurse burnout and job dissatisfaction. *Journal of the American Medical Association, 288*(16), 1987–1993.

Aiken, L., Havens, D., & Sloane, D. (2000). The Magnet Services Recognition Program: A comparison to two groups of Magnet hospitals. *American Journal of Nursing, 100*(3), 26–35.

Aiken, L. H., Lake, E. T., Sochalski, J., & Sloane, D. M. (1997). Design of an outcomes study of the organization of hospital AIDS care. *Research in the Sociology of Health Care, 14*, 3–26.

Aiken, L. H. & Sloane, D. M. (1997a). Effects of organizational innovations in AIDS care on burnout among urban hospital nurses. *Work and Occupations, 24*(4), 453–477.

Aiken, L. H. & Sloane, D. M. (1997b). Effects of specialization and client differentiation on the status of nurses: The case of AIDS. *Journal of Health and Social Behavior, 38*(September), 203–222.

Aiken, L. H., Sloane, D. M., & Klocinski, J. L. (1997). Hospital nurses' occupational exposure to blood, prospective, retrospective, and institutional reports. *American Journal of Public Health, 87*(1), 103–107.

Aiken, L. H., Sloane, D. M., & Lake, E. T. (1997). Satisfaction with inpatient AIDS care: A national comparison of dedicated units and scattered beds. *Medical Care, 36*(9), 948–962.

Aiken, L. H., Sloane, D. M., Lake, E. T, Sochalski, J., & Weber, A. L. (1999). Organization and outcomes of inpatient AIDS care. *Medical Care, 37*(8), 760–772.

Aiken, L. H., Smith, H. L., & Lake, E. T. (1994). Lower Medicare mortality rates among a set of hospitals known for good nursing care. *Medical Care, 32*(8), 771–787.

Aiken, L. H., Sochalski, J., & Lake, E. T. (1997). Studying outcomes of organizational change in health services. *Medical Care, 35*(suppl), NS6–N18.

American Hospital Association. (2007). *The 2007 state of America's hospitals—Taking the pulse.* Retrieved from http://www.aha.org/aha/content/2007/PowerPoint/StateofHospitalsChartPack2007.ppt

American Nurses Credentialing Center. (2010). *Magnet characteristics.* Retrieved from http://www.nursecredentialing.org/Magnet/ProgramOverview/Magnet-Characteristics.aspx

Armstrong, K. J. & Laschinger, H. (2006). Structural empowerment: Magnet hospital characteristics and patient safety culture: Making the link. *Journal of Nursing Care Quality, 21*(2), 124–132.

Armstrong, K. J., Laschinger, H., & Wong, C. (2009). Workplace empowerment and Magnet hospital characteristics as predictors of patient safety climate. *Journal of Nursing Care Quality, 24*(1):55-62.

Bates, D. W., Pruess, K., & Platt, R. (1995). Serious falls in hospitalized patients: Correlates and resource utilization. *American Journal of Medicine, 99*(2), 137–143.

Beckrich, K. & Aronovitch, S. A. (1999). Hospital-acquired pressure ulcers: A comparison of costs of medical and surgical patients. *Nursing Economic$, 17*(5), 263–271.

Berquist-Beringer, S., Davidson, J., Agosto, C., Linde, N. K., Abel, M., Spurling, K., Dunton, N., & Christopher, A. (2009). Evaluation of the National Database of Nursing Quality Indicators (NDNQI) training program on pressure ulcers. *Journal of Continuing Education in Nursing, 40*(6), 252–260.

Brady-Schwartz, D. C. (2005). Further evidence on the Magnet Recognition Program: Implications for nursing leaders. *Journal of Nursing Administration, 35*(9), 397–403.

Cimmiotti, P., Quinlan, P., Larson, E., Pastor, D., & Stone, P. (2005). The nursing process and perceived work environment of nurses. *Nursing Research, 54*(6), 384–390.

Clarke, S. P., Sloane, D. M., & Aiken, L. H. (2002). Effects of hospital staffing and organizational climate on needle-stick injuries to nurses. *American Journal of Public Health, 92*(7), 1115–1119.

Dall, T. M., Chen, Y. J., Seifert, R. F., Maddox, P. J., & Hogan, P. F. (2009). The economic value of professional nursing. *Medical Care, 47*(1), 97–104

DeSilets, L. & Pinkerton, S. E. (2005). Administrative angles: The financial return on Magnet recognition. *Journal of Continuing Education in Nursing, 36*(2), 51–52.

Doloresco, L. G. (2004). Building a business case for Magnet designation in VHA. Retrieved from http://www1.va.gov/nursing/docs/FinalBusCasereport11-26.pdf

Dunton, N., Gajewski, B., Klaus, S., & Pierson, P. (2007). The relationship of nursing workforce characteristics to patient outcomes: A study to assess the economic value of nursing staff and registered nurses. Retrieved from www.medscape.com/viewarticle/569394_4

Dunton, N, Gajewski, B., Taunton, R. L., & Moore, J. (2004). Nursing staffing and patient falls in acute care hospital units. *Nursing Outlook, 52*(1), 53–59.

Gardner, J. K., Fogg, L., Thomas-Hawkins, C., & Latham, C. E. (2007). The relationships between nurses' perceptions of the hemodialysis work environment and nurse turnover, patient satisfaction, and hospitalizations. *Nephrology Nursing Journal, 34*(3), 271–281.

Gelinas, L. & Bohlen, C. (2002). Tomorrow's work force: A strategic approach. Irving, TX: VHA Research Series.

Goode, C., & Blegen, M. (2009). The link between nurse staffing and patient outcomes. Abstract and presentation at National Magnet Conference, Louisville, KY, Oct 1–3.

Hassmiller, S. B., & Christopher, M. A. (2009). Making the business case for nursing to the business community and to CEOs. *Nurse Leader, 7*(2), 48–52.

Havens, D. S. (2001). Comparing nursing infrastructure and outcomes: ANCC Magnet and non-Magnet CNE's report. *Nursing Economic$, 19*(6), 258–266.

Havens, D. S. & Aiken, L. H. (1999). Shaping systems to promote desired outcomes: the Magnet hospital model. *Journal of Nursing Administration, 29*(2), 14–20.

Havens, D. S., & Johnston, M. A. (2004). Achieving Magnet recognition: Chief nurse executives and Magnet coordinators tell their stories. *Journal of Nursing Administration, 34*(12), 579–588.

Hines, P. A., & Yu, K. M. (2009). The changing reimbursement landscape: Nurses' role in quality and operational excellence. *Nursing Economic$, 27*(1), 1–7.

Hitcho, E. B., Krauss, M. J., Birges, Claiborne-Dunagan, W., Fischer, I., Johnson, S., Nast, P. A., et al. (2004). Characteristics and circumstances of falls in hospital setting: A prospective analysis. *Journal of General Internal Medicine, 19*(7), 732–739.

Hook, M. L., & Winchel, S. (2006). Fall-related injuries in acute care: Reducing the risk of harm. *MEDSURG Nursing, 15*(6), 370–381.

How to refocus your projects into value. Retrieved from www.valuedeliverymanagement.net/Portals/0/download/h2_ref_proj_on_value.pdf

Hughes, L., Chang, Y., & Mark, B. (2009). Quality and strength of patient safety climate on medical surgical units. *Health Care Management Review, 34*(1), 19–28.

Jagger, J., Hunt, E. H., & Peatson, R. D. (1990). Estimated cost of needle-stick for six major needled devices. *Infection Control and Hospital Epidemiology, 11*(11), 584–588.

Jones, C. B. & Gates, M. (2007). The cost and benefits of nurse turnover: A business case for nurse retention. *Online Journal of Issues in Nursing, 12*(3). Retrieved from http://www.nursingworld.org/MainMenuCategories/ANAMarketplace/ANAPeriodicals/OJIN/TableofContents/Volume122007/No3Sept07/NurseRetention.aspx

Kramer, M. (1990). The Magnet hospitals: Excellence revisited. *Journal of Nursing Administration, 20*(9), 35–44.

Kramer, M. & Schmalenberg, C. E. (1988a). Magnet hospitals I: Institutions of excellence. *Journal of Nursing Administration, 18*(1), 13–24.

Kramer, M. & Schmalenberg, C. E. (1988b). Magnet hospitals II: Institutions of excellence. Journal of Nursing Administration, 18(2), 11–19.

Lacey, S. R., Cox, K. S., Lorfing, K. C., Teasley, S. L., Carroll, C. A., & Sexton, K. (2007). Nursing support, workload, and intent to stay in Magnet, Magnet-aspiring, and non-Magnet hospitals. *Journal of Nursing Administration, 37*(4), 199–205.

Laschinger, H. K., Almost, L., & Tuer-Hodes, D. (2003). Workplace empowerment and Magnet hospital characteristics: Making the link. *Journal of Nursing Administration, 33*(7/8), 410–422.

Laschinger, H., Finegan, J. E., Shamian, J., & Wilk, P. (2004). A longitudinal analysis of the impact of workplace empowerment on work satisfaction. *Journal of Organizational Behavior, 25*(4), 527–545.

Laschinger, H., & Leiter, M. P. (2006). The impact of nursing work environments on patient safety outcomes: The mediating role of burnout/engagement. *Journal of Nursing Administration, 36*(5), 259–267.

Laschinger. H., Shamian, J., & Thomson, D. (2001). Impact of Magnet hospital characteristics on nurses' perceptions of trust, burnout, quality of care, and work satisfaction. *Nursing Economic$, 19*(5), 209–219.

Lavizzo-Mourey, R., & Verplanck, J. (2009, July 2). Recession is making nursing shortage worse. *The Philadelphia Inquirer.*

McClure, M. L., Poulin, M., Sovie, M., & Wandell, M. (1983). *Magnet hospitals: Attraction and retention of professional nurses.* Kansas City, MO: American Nurses Association.

McConnell, C. R. (1999). Staff turnover: occasional friend, frequent foe, a frustration. *Health Care Manager, 18*(1), 1–13.

Mills, A. (2008). Effect of Magnet recognition presentation on patient outcomes. Abstract and Presentation, National Magnet Conference, Salt Lake City, October 15–17.

Neisner, J., & Raymond, B. (2002). Nursing staffing and care delivery models: a review of the evidence. Retrieved from http://www.kpihp.org/kpihp/CMS/Files/nurse_staffing.pdf

Nelson, A., Matz, M., Chen, F., Siddharthan, K., Lloyd, J., & Fragala, G. (2006). Development and evaluation of a multifaceted ergonomics program to prevent injuries associated with patient handling tasks. *International Journal of Nursing Studies, 43*, 717–733.

Nurmi, I., & Luthje, P. (2002). Incidence and costs of falls and fall injuries among elderly in institutional care. *Scandinavian Journal of Primary Health Care, 20*(2), 118–122.

Poduska, D. D. (2005). Magnet designation in a community hospital. *Nursing Adminstration Quarterly, 29*(3), 223–227.

Potter, P., Barr, N., McSweeney, M., & Sledge, J. (2003). Identifying nurse staffing and patient outcome relationships: A guide for change in care delivery. *Nursing Economic$, 21*(4), 158–166.

Prosci. (2009, 2010). *Business case toolkit.* Retrieved from www.prosci.com/t3-toc.htm

Robert Wood Johnson Foundation. (2009). *Charting nursing's future. Nursing prescription for a reformed health system: Use exemplary nursing initiatives to expand access, improve quality, reduce costs, and promote prevention.* Retrieved from http://www.rwjf.org/files/research/200904 08chartingnursing9.pdf

Rondeau, K. V., & Wagar, T. H. (2006). Nurse and resident satisfaction in Magnet long-term care organizations: do high involvement approaches matter? *Journal of Nursing Management, 14*(3), 244–250.

Rosenberg, M. C. (2009). Do Magnet-recognized hospitals provide better care? Presentation, National Magnet Conference, Louisville, KY, October 1–3.

Sandhusen, A., Rusynko, B., Wethington, N. (2004). Return on investment for a peri-operative nurse fellowship. *AORN Journal, 80*(1), 73–81.

Schmalenberg, C., & Kramer, M. (2008). Essentials of a productive nurse work environment. *Nursing Research, 57*(1), 2–13.

Scott, J. G., Sochalski. J., & Aiken, L. (1999). Review of Magnet hospital research: Findings and implications for professional nursing practice. *Journal of Nursing Administration, 29*(1), 9–19.

Shorr, R. I., Mion, L. C., Chandler, M. A., Rosenblatt, L. C., Lynch, D., & Kessler, L. A. (2008). Improving the capture of fall events in hospitals: Combining a service for evaluating patient falls with an incident reporting system. *Journal of the American Geriatrics Society, 56*(4), 701–704.

Smith, H., Tallman, R., & Kelley, K. (2006). Magnet hospital characteristics and northern Canadian nurses' job satisfaction. *Canadian Journal of Nursing Leadership, 19*(3), 73–86.

Stone, P. W., & Gershon, R. R. M. (2006). Nurse work environments and occupational safety in intensive care units. *Policy, Politics, & Nursing Practice, 7*(4), 240–247.

Stone, P. W., Mooney-Kane, K., Larson, E. L., Horan, T., Glance, L. G., Zwanziger, J., & Dick, A. W. (2007). Nurse working conditions and patient safety outcomes. *Medical Care, 45*(6), 571–578.

The Advisory Board Company. (2000). *Reversing the flight of talent: Nursing retention in an era of gathering shortage.* Washington, DC: The Advisory Board Company.

Tigert, J. A., & Laschinger, H. K. (2004). Critical care nurses' perceptions of workplace empowerment, Magnet hospital traits and mental health. *Dynamics, 15*(4), 19–23.

Tuazon, N. (2007). Is Magnet a money-maker? *Nursing Management, 38*(6), 24–30.

Ulrich, B. T., Buerhaus, P. I., Donelan, K., Norman, L., & Dittus, R. (2007). Magnet status and registered nurse views of the work environment and nursing as a career. *Journal of Nursing Administration, 37*(5), 212–220.

Unruh, L. (2008). Nursing staffing and patient, nurse and financial outcomes. *American Journal of Nursing, 108*(1), 62–72.

Upenieks, V. (2003a). The interrelationship of organizational characteristics of Magnet hospitals, nursing leadership, and nursing job satisfaction. *Health Care Manager, 22*(2), 83–98.

Upenieks, V. (2003b). Recruitment and retention strategies: A Magnet hospital prevention model. *Nursing Economic$, 21*(1), 7–13, 23.

Upenieks, V. (2003c). What constitutes effective leadership? Perceptions of Magnet and non-Magnet nurse leaders. *Journal of Nursing Administration, 33*(9), 456–467.

Value Delivery Management. (2009). *The VDM business case generation program.* Retrieved from http://www.valuedeliverymanagement.com/pages/The-VDM-Business-Case-Generation-Program.html

VHA. (2002). *The business case for workforce stability.* Retrieved from http://www.healthleadersmedia.com/content/132674.pdf

Waldman, J. D., Kelly, F., Arora, S., & Smith, H. L. (2004). The shocking cost of turnover in healthcare. *Health Care Manage Rev, 29*(1), 2–7.

Weaver, D. J., & Sorrell-Jones, J. (2007). The business case as a strategic tool for change. *Journal of Nursing Administration, 37*(9), 414–419.

Wilburn, S. Q. (2004). Needle-stick and sharps injury prevention. *Online Journal of Issures in Nursing, 9*(3). Retrieved from http://www.nursingworld.org/MainMenuCategories/ANAMarketplace/ANAPeriodicals/OJIN/TableofContents/Volume92004/No3Sept04/InjuryPrevention.aspx

Wolf, G., Triolo, P., & Reid-Ponte, P., (2008). Magnet recognition program: The next generation. *Journal of Nursing Administration, 38*(4), 200–204.

Woods, D. K. (2002a). Realizing your marketing influence Part 1: Meeting patient needs through collaboration. *Journal of Nursing Administration, 32*(4), 189–195.

Woods, D. K. (2002b). Realizing your marketing influence Part 3: Professional certification as a marketing tool. *Journal of Nursing Administration, 32*(7/8), 379–386.

Woods, D. K., & Cardin, S. (2002). Realizing your marketing influence Part 2: Marketing from the inside out. *Journal of Nursing Administration, 32*(6): 323-30.

Implications for Health Policy

Stephanie L. Ferguson, PhD, RN, FAAN
Karen Drenkard, PhD, RN, NEA-BC, FAAN
Mary Jo Assi, MS, RN, APRN-BC, AHN-BC
Yasmin Kazzaz, MHA

Nursing would be best positioned to influence the future shape of health care if it combines its quest for holistic and patient-centered care with science-based advocacy and evidence-based skepticism about any kind of reform that does not fundamentally change the organization and culture of health care.
Linda Aiken, *Policy, Politics, & Nursing Practice, 2008*

INTRODUCTION

The U.S. healthcare system is badly in need of reform, with vast and daunting challenges. The current system is fragmented and constantly changing because of a variety of issues. These include fluctuating healthcare financing from rising healthcare costs; an increase in medical errors and a decrease in patient safety and quality care; changing demographics, including a growing aging population; an increase in chronic diseases and how they are managed; workforce shortages and imbalances; and millions of under- and uninsured citizens. Efforts of the Obama administration to pass a major health reform agenda have far-reaching implications.

To strengthen healthcare delivery and move toward a more preferred state, individuals and organizations are calling for increased patient safety and quality initiatives; a resurgence and strengthening of primary care and the infrastructure to support it; aggressive strategies to reduce healthcare costs and increase access; the development and sustainability of positive work environments; and improved recruitment, retention, and re-education of healthcare workers to ensure continued competency.

Health policy, given its inherent complexity, will continue to evolve (Longest, 2006), and it is imperative that nurses be at the forefront. Nurses must be leaders in promoting healthcare reform and patient-centric health policies that make a difference in people's lives, communities, societies, the nation, and the world. To understand the role of nursing in health policy development and its importance in the context of Magnet® recognition, one must understand what health policies are and how they are developed. This chapter will examine the public policy making process, the role of the Magnet nurse in health policy, and implications for the future.

HOW HEALTH POLICIES ARE DEVELOPED

Health policies are public policies determined by regulators, legislators, and judicial and governmental entities to promote the health of citizens. Health policy decisions and changes are driven by access, cost, and quality. Therefore, in health policy debate and reform, arguments for or against usually focus on one of these areas:

- How many people will have *access*?
- How much will this *cost* individuals and society?
- What are the *quality* measures, metrics, and outcomes, including performance?

The policy process, whether it is health, social, or public, is often divided into three phases: policy formulation; policy implementation; and policy evaluation, feedback, and modification. Longest (2006) describes policy formulation as the phase where problems, solutions, and political circumstances are brought to the table. He further notes that timing is critical and agenda setting should be considered when a window of opportunity opens. The circumstances should be such that key players and stakeholders can come together, agree to disagree, and work to develop changes or policies that are the preferred way forward.

Once legislation is written and formally enacted, the policy implementation phase begins and rules are determined to operationalize the enacted legislation. This phase determines the policy that will be operationalized by law. The policy modification phase allows for feedback and changes to previous decisions made during the formulation and implementation phases.

Longest's perspective on public policy making in the United States appears straightforward and linear, but he reminds us that external forces influence policy making. Special interest groups, individuals, organizations, and political entities all have an impact. Therefore, health policy development and implementation are political and imperfect in most instances. He argues that one must be competent in the policy process to shape the policy environments of health services. This competence is especially crucial for nurse leaders so they can spearhead effective strategic management in healthcare organizations. Policy competency helps chief nurses and nurse managers anticipate and lead their hospitals' response to "the opportunities and threats emanating from their policy environments" (Longest, 2004, p. 71).

THE ROLE OF MAGNET NURSES IN HEALTH POLICY

In Magnet hospitals, nurses have higher education levels and greater participation in decision-making. As such, they are positioned to serve as leaders to influence healthcare policy development and implementation. There is a growing body of research sustained over a decade that indicates positive outcomes in Magnet hospitals. The evidence includes positive nursing practice environments that lower rates of mortality and failure to rescue (Aiken, Clarke, Sloane et al., 2008). There also is evidence that Magnet hospitals' characteristics and work environments improve clinical outcomes such as decreasing mortality, patient falls, and pressure ulcers (Aiken, Havens, & Sloane, 2000; Lundmark, 2008).

The Magnet Vision

Magnet organizations will serve as the fount of knowledge and expertise for the delivery of nursing care globally. They will be solidly grounded in core Magnet principles, flexible, and constantly striving for discovery and innovation. They will lead the reformation of health care; the discipline of nursing; and care of the patient, family, and community.
The Commission on Magnet Recognition, 2008
Source: ANCC, 2008

Nurses are essential to ensure quality health care that is safe, accessible, and affordable. Magnet nurses possess leadership and policy skills that ensure patient safety and quality healthcare delivery (Armstrong & Laschinger 2006). They are empowered to communicate more effectively and contribute successfully to safe patient care. Magnet nurses create practice environments that positively influence the climate of patient safety (Armstrong, Laschinger, & Wong, 2009; Hughes, Chang, & Mark, 2009; Schmalenberg & Kramer, 2008; Stone, Mooney, Larson et al., 2007).

Magnet nurses are competent political players and key stakeholders in health policy development and implementation. They are in a unique position to make sustainable healthcare changes and continuously improve health outcomes because of the nature of their leadership capacity, innovative spirits, knowledge, skills, and abilities. Magnet nurses lead the way in determining solutions and best practices in the quest for affordable and accessible health care for all. This is reflected in the Magnet Recognition Program®'s vision. (*See* The Magnet Vision.)

One nurse, a member of the American Academy of Nursing, summarized the power of the Magnet movement. Attaining voluntary Magnet recognition, she says, has raised the bar on safety and quality at her hospital in a way that no federal regulation, external regulatory requirements, or state health agency standard has been able to accomplish in the past 20 years (Personal Communication, Academy of Nursing Magnet Expert Panel Meeting, November 2009, Atlanta, GA).

IMPLICATIONS FOR HEALTH POLICY

What are the implications for health policy that can tap into this Magnet movement and spread to all healthcare organizations in the United States and possibly the world? And how can policy recommendations aid in creating a preferred future for delivery systems that improve quality, contain costs, and provide healthcare access to our communities?

The original Magnet research was conducted to address the national problem of high nursing turnover and vacancy rates in the acute-care setting (McClure et al., 1983). Additional data link Magnet status to improved clinical outcomes (Aiken, Havens, & Sloane, 2000; Brady-Schwartz, 2005), and lower vacancy and turnover rates (Upenieks, 2005). Some studies indicate that the Magnet Recognition Program has been successful in improving the work environment for nurses, as best characterized by Lacey, Cox et al. (2007). This positive work environment is necessary because turnover of registered nurses destabilizes the economy of health care. The costs of care are steadily increasing, and salary expenditures in hospitals are the largest percentage of expense. The high costs of recruitment, orientation, and training of new employees add to these expenses. Any strategy that will lower RN turnover deserves attention from policy makers. They should consider several key implications for the policy arena.

INCREASE RESEARCH FUNDING

The first policy implication is to increase research funding dedicated to better understanding Magnet as an innovative program that helps create stable work environments through controlling antecedents to turnover. Pilot program research can examine ways to expedite the process and disseminate and apply best practices found in Magnet facilities. Leadership models based on Transformational Leadership characteristics should be developed to allow for control over the antecedent variables. Research funding should include interventional strategies that explore the most effective leadership models, such as those in Magnet facilities that reduce RN turnover. Pilot sites should be identified, and outcome measurements shared.

Magnet hospitals serve as examples of stable work environments, and increased research is needed into the predictive variables that are essential to sustainability of excellence in patient care outcomes. Magnet requirements, based on the work of nurses, are increasingly linked to positive patient care outcomes (Lundmark, 2008). Further research is necessary to determine the essential elements of structures and processes that must be in place to reach excellent clinical outcomes. Once identified, these essential elements cannot be ignored or removed when cost pressures escalate. Research into the positive impact of Magnet recognition and which Sources of Evidence most positively impact work environments would help focus improvement efforts. The benefits to nurses as caregivers and patients as care receivers in Magnet facilities affect the community, and further research is indicated.

INCENTIVE PAY FOR LOW RN TURNOVER

The second policy recommendation is for Medicare pay-for-performance standards to include incentive pay for hospitals that demonstrate lower RN turnover. Pay-for-performance recognizes and financially motivates care providers to reach certain outcome measures. Research links investment in nursing with better patient outcomes (Aiken, 2008). Therefore, pay-for-performance initiatives could improve nursing processes and structures in hospitals.

The Medicare Payment Advisory Commission (*Quality Letter* lead story, 2005) has called for the consideration and creation of quality incentive payment policies for hospitals. Considerable attention has been paid to the development of national policies that address performance measurement, public reporting, and "value-based" purchasing (Kurtzman, Dawson, & Johnson, 2008). Nurses are key change agents in improvement of quality and safety. Bedside nurses in a positive work environment are a foundational element for these improvement efforts.

RN turnover as a specific outcome measure should be considered as one of hospitals' quality measures in this plan. Rewards to hospitals can include bonus payments, higher reimbursement rates, and public recognition. It is important that quality improvement plans to reduce nursing turnover be evidence-based, so as to include research on Magnet hospitals in the array of tactical considerations for improving nursing turnover (Cummings & McLennan, 2005). The Centers for Medicare and Medicaid Services (CMS) could include proposals linking leadership and nursing turnover in their demonstration projects to assess quality performance and improvement. Hospitals that achieve Magnet recognition should be eligible for improved rates of reimbursement as long as they maintain that status. Magnet standards require that nursing-sensitive data, patient satisfaction, and RN satisfaction be in the upper half of benchmarked results for at least two years.

Magnet status now serves as recognition of higher-performing healthcare organizations. Federal incentive programs should motivate and financially reward hospitals that achieve Magnet status. Research (Lacey, Cox, Lorfing et al., 2007) reveals that staff nurses at Magnet hospitals are less likely to quit. Lower turnover rates mean lower costs. Financial incentives would encourage more hospitals to meet Magnet criteria—not only improving the stability of the workforce, but improving patient outcomes as well.

STANDARDIZE DATA

Another policy implication that arises from the Magnet Recognition Program is the need to standardize the data elements collected across the nation. Currently there are multiple sets of data, definitions, indicators, and measures in patient satisfaction, nurse satisfaction, and clinical outcomes. While the National Quality Foundation (NQF) and Hospital Consumer Assessment of Healthcare Providers and Systems (HCAHPS) have made some progress in this area, there are still obstacles to standardizing comparative data. With standard data sets, vendors could develop survey instruments that use the same criteria, which would improve comparative review. Once the data were reported nationally, healthcare consumers could make informed decisions about where to receive care. This is the foundation of the quality improvement process and transparency in reporting outcome results.

HEALTHCARE WORKFORCE BENEFITS

There are implications for the healthcare workforce as well. Research has demonstrated that positive work environments lead to improved occupational safety in the clinical environment, including occupational injuries, musculoskeletal injuries, and needle-sticks (Stone & Gershon, 2006). In particular, Magnet hospitals had significantly lower rates in all three occupational health outcomes, and less exposure to blood and body fluids.

The health workforce requires an adequate supply of nurses. Solving the nursing shortage and decreasing turnover are national and global priorities (Buchan & Aiken, 2008). The Health Resources and Services Administration (HRSA) offers grants that must be continued and extended, such as the 2002 Nurse Reinvestment Act, which included provisions for grants to encourage facilities to implement Magnet strategies (Collins, Davis, & Lambrew, 2004).

LEADING THE WAY

Nursing as a discipline—composed of more than three million RNs in the United States—is well positioned to influence the future of patient care delivery. It should come as no surprise that nurses want to work in an environment that encourages their professional development, promotes quality improvement and safety, and focuses on the patient. The Magnet Recognition Program is emerging as a community of practitioners leading the way in the reformation of care delivery. Great nursing leaders working in great structures develop extraordinary professional practice models. This, in turn, leads to new knowledge, innovation, and superior patient outcomes. The Magnet Recognition Program continues to raise the bar for nursing excellence in patient care.

REFERENCES

All URLs retrieved September 12, 2010.

Aiken, L. H. (2008). Economics of nursing. *Policy, Politics, & Nursing Practice. 9*(2), 73–79.

Aiken, L. H., Clarke, S., Sloane D., Lake, E., & Cheney, T. (2008). Effects of hospital care environment on patient mortality and nurse outcomes. *Journal of Nursing Administration, 38*(5), 223–229.

Aiken, L. H., Havens, D. S., & Sloane, D. M. (2009). The Magnet nursing services recognition program: a comparison of two groups of Magnet hospitals. *Journal of Nursing Administration, 39*(7/8 Suppl), S5–S14.

American Nurses Credentialing Center. (2008). *Application manual: Magnet Recognition Program, 2008.,* Silver Spring, MD: Author.

Armstrong, K., & Laschinger, H. (2006). Structural empowerment, Magnet hospital characteristics, and patient safety culture: making the link. *Journal of Nursing Care Quality, 21*(2), 124–132.

Armstrong, K., Laschinger, H., & Wong, C. (2009). Workplace empowerment and Magnet hospital characteristics as predictors of patient safety climate. Journal of Nursing Care Quality, 24(1), 55–62.

Brady-Schwartz, D. C. (2005). Further evidence on the Magnet recognition program: Implications for nursing leaders. *Journal of Nursing Administration, 35*(9), 397–403.

Buchan, J., & Aiken, L. H. (2008). Solving nursing shortages: a common priority. *Journal of Clinical Nursing, 17*(24), 3262–3268.

Collins, S. R., Davis, K., & Lambrew, J. M. (2004). Healthcare reform returns to the national agenda: 2004 Presidential candidates proposals. (October 8.) New York: The Commonwealth Fund. Retrieved Septemeber 12, 2010 from http://www.cmwf.org/publications/publications_show. htm?doc_id=221448

Cummings, G., & McLennan, M. (2005). Advanced practice nursing: Leadership to effect policy change. *Journal of Nursing Administration, 35*(2), 61–66.

Hughes, L., Chang, Y., & Mark, B. (2009). Quality and strength of patient safety climate on medical-surgical units. *Health Care Management Review. 34*(1), 19–28.

Kurtzman, E. T., Dawson, E. M., & Johnson, J. E. (2008). The current state of nursing performance measurement, public reporting, and value-based purchasing. *Policy, Politics, & Nursing Practice, 9*(3), 181–191.

Lacey, S. R., Cox, K. S., Lorfing, K. C., Teasley, S. L., Carroll, C. A., & Sexton, K. (2007). Nursing support, workload, and intent to stay in Magnet, Magnet-aspiring, and non-Magnet hospitals. *Journal of Nursing Administration, 37*(4), 199–205.

Longest, B. (2004). An international constant: The crucial role of policy competence in the effective strategic management of health services organizations. *Health Services Management Research, 17*(2), 71–78.

Longest, B. (2006). Health policymaking in the United States. Chicago, IL: Health Administration Press.

Lundmark, V. (2008). Magnet environments for professional nursing practice. In R. G. Hughes (Ed.), Patient safety and quality: An evidence-based handbook for nurses. Rockville, MD: Agency for HealthCare Research and Quality.

McClure, M. L., Poulin, M. A., Sovie, M. D., & Wandell, M. A. (1983). Magnet hospitals: Attraction and retention of professional nurses. Kansas City, MO: American Nurses Association.

Quality Letter (QL) lead story. (2005). Changing the dial on quality: What will pay-for-performance reimbursement strategies mean for providing better care? *Quality Letter for Healthcare Leaders, 17*(4), 2–8.

Schmalenberg, C., & Kramer, M., (2008). Essentials of a productive nurse work environment. *Nursing Research, 57*(1), 2–13.

Stone, P. W., & Gershon, R. R. M. (2006). Nurse work environments and occupational safety in intensive care units, *Policy, Politics, & Nursing Practice, 7*(4), 240–247.

Stone, P., Mooney-Kane, C., Larson, E. L., Horan, T., Glance, L. G., Zwanziger, J., & Dick, A. W. (2007). Nurse working conditions and patient safety outcomes. *Medical Care, 45*(6), 571–578.

Ulrich, B. T., Buerhaus, P., Donelan, K., Norman, L., and Dittus, R. (2007). Magnet status and registered nurse views of the work environment and nursing as a career. *Journal of Nursing Administration, 37*(5), 212-220.

Upenieks, V. (2003). Recruitment and retention strategies: a Magnet hospital prevention model. *Nursing Economics, 21*(1), 7–13, 23.

Upenieks, V. (2005). Recruitment and retention strategies: A Magnet hospital prevention model. MEDSURG Nursing (Apr Suppl), 21-27.

Index

Made in the USA
Middletown, DE
11 February 2015